Managing bipolar disorder in clinical practice

Third edition

Managing bipolar disorder in clinical practice
Third edition

Editor
Eduard Vieta
Director of the Bipolar Disorders Program
Hospital Clinic
University of Barcelona
Spain

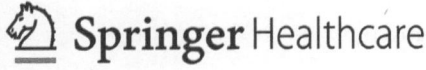

Published by Springer Healthcare Ltd, 236 Gray's Inn Road, London, WC1X 8HB, UK.

www.springerhealthcare.com

© 2013 Springer Healthcare, a part of Springer Science+Business Media.

First edition 2007
Second edition 2009
Third edition 2013

British Library Cataloguing-in-Publication Data.

A catalogue record for this book is available from the British Library.

ISBN 978-1-908517-73-9

Project editor: Katrina Dorn
Designer: Joe Harvey
Artworker: Sissan Mollerfors
Production: Marina Maher
Printed in Great Britain by Latimer Trend and Co. Ltd.

Contents

Author biography

Professor Eduard Vieta is Professor of Psychiatry, Head of Department, and the Director of the Bipolar Disorders Program in the Hospital Clinic at the University of Barcelona, Catalonia, Spain. He is the current Director of the Bipolar Research Program at the Spanish Research Network on Mental Diseases (CIBERSAM), funded by the Spanish Ministry of Science and Innovation. His research focuses on the neurobiology, epidemiology, and treatment of bipolar disorder. Professor Vieta received the Aristotle award in 2005, the Mogens Schou award in 2007, and the Colvin Price on Outstanding Achievement in Mood Disorders Research by the Brain and Behaviour Research Foundation in 2012. He has made significant contributions to many of the major published bipolar disorder treatment guidelines and has authored more than 450 original articles, 200 book chapters, and 27 complete books. His H index is 57 and he has over 12,000 citations. Furthermore, he is on the editorial board of a range of international scientific journals. He has served as an invited professor at Harvard University and as neuroscience scientific advisor to the European Presidency.

Chapter 1

Overview of bipolar disorder

Definitions

Bipolar disorder is a severe chronic mood disorder characterized by episodes of mania or hypomania alternating or commingling with episodes of depression. Bipolar disorder may also be referred to as manic depression, bipolar affective disorder, or bipolar spectrum disorder.

There are two main diagnostic schemes defining bipolar disorder: the *International Classification of Disease* of the World Health Organization (10th revision; ICD-10) [1,2] and the *Diagnostic and Statistical Manual of Mental Disorders* of the American Psychiatric Association (4th edition, text revisions; DSM-IV-TR) [3]. A new edition of the DSM is scheduled for 2013 and a new edition of the ICD is scheduled for 2015.

ICD-10 definition

The ICD-10 defines bipolar affective disorder as follows [1,2]: a disorder characterized by two or more episodes in which the patient's mood and activity levels are significantly disturbed, this disturbance consisting on some occasions of an elevation of mood and increased energy and activity (hypomania or mania) and on others of a lowering of mood and decreased energy and activity (depression). Repeated episodes of hypomania or mania only are classified as bipolar.

The ICD-10 definition includes the following subdivisions that reflect the nature of the current episode:

- hypomania;
- mania without psychotic symptoms;

E. Vieta, *Managing Bipolar Disorder in Clinical Practice*,
DOI: 10.1007/978-1-908517-94-4_1, © Springer Healthcare 2013

- mania with psychotic symptoms;
- mild or moderate depression;
- severe depression without psychotic symptoms;
- severe depression with psychotic symptoms;
- mixed;
- in remission; and
- unspecified.

DSM-IV-TR definition

According to DSM-IV-TR, bipolar disorder is defined as the occurrence of even a single period of mood elevation not attributable to substance abuse or a general medical condition [3]. The definition does not include age of onset or course of illness as diagnostic criteria.

DSM-IV-TR includes four categories in the bipolar spectrum that reflect the types of episodes that have occurred over an individual's lifetime:

1. Bipolar disorder type I: at least one manic or mixed episode; major depressive episodes (MDEs) typical but not required.
2. Bipolar disorder type II: at least one hypomanic episode and at least one MDE; no manic or mixed episodes.
3. Cyclothymic disorder: long-term depressive and hypomanic symptoms; no major depression or mania.
4. Bipolar disorder not otherwise specified: manic symptoms but criteria not met for bipolar I, bipolar II, or cyclothymia; depressive symptoms not required.

DSM-IV-TR includes the following categories for defining the current episode:

- manic;
- major depressive;
- mixed state;
- hypomanic;
- cyclothymia;
- rapid cycling; and
- not otherwise specified.

Clinical and diagnostic features associated with the ICD-10 and DSM-IV-TR criteria are discussed in further detail in Chapter 4.

Types of mood episode

Mania

Mania is a complex mood state characterized by a rapid and major change in the individual's usual behavior. Mania has a diverse clinical presentation; a constellation of symptoms, lasting for at least 1 week, is required for diagnosis. The range of symptoms in mania has been described by Goodwin and Jamison and is summarized in Table 1.1 [4].

Mania is sometimes subdivided into euphoric mania (with expansivity and elation) and irritable mania (with anger, aggressiveness, or even furor). Alternatively, mania may be distinguished by the presence of psychotic features (such as hallucinations, delusions, formal thought disorder, catatonia, or agitations). Moreover, delusions can be 'mood congruent' (eg, grandiosity) or 'mood incongruent' (eg, persecutory, strange delusions).

Hypomania

Hypomania is an attenuated form of mania that by definition is not associated with psychosis or delusions. It refers to a clearly abnormal mood state with mild-to-moderate symptoms of mania that may last for a few days or for many months. The key distinctions from mania are that hypomania can be diagnosed after 4 days and, although the disorder is associated with an unequivocal change in functioning, there is no marked impairment, at least according to DSM-IV-TR.

The limits of hypomania are quite vague and it may be difficult to distinguish hypomania from the person's usual behavior; this is often the case with hyperthymic personality. Consequently, hypomania is often undiagnosed. For some patients, hypomania is a pleasant state of good humor and high productivity. For most people, however, hypomanic symptoms, even lasting under 4 days, can be problematic. Things said or done during a hypomanic episode often have negative long-term consequences. Hypomania may also be a prelude to a full manic episode or a severe depression. Although DSM-IV-TR explicitly excludes the possibility of diagnosing mixed hypomanic episodes, such episodes exist and may be difficult to treat [5].

Manic episodes: mean rate of symptom occurrence

Symptom	Occurrence (%)
Mood symptoms	
Irritability	80
Euphoria	71
Depression	72
Lability	69
Expansiveness	60
Cognitive symptoms	
Grandiosity	78
Flight of ideas, racing thoughts	71
Distractibility, poor concentration	71
Confusion	25
Psychotic symptoms	
Any delusion	48
Grandiosity	47
Persecutory paranoid	28
Passivity	15
Any hallucinations	15
Auditory hallucinations	18
Visual hallucinations	10
Olfactory hallucinations	17
History of psychotic symptoms	58
Thought disorder	19
First rank symptoms (Schneider)	18
Activity and behavior during mania	
Hyperactivity	87
Decreased sleep	81
Violent assaultive behavior	49
Rapid pressured speech	98
Hyperverbosity	89
Nudity, sexual exposure	29
Hypersexuality	57
Extravagance	55
Religiosity	39
Head decoration	34
Regression (pronounced)	28
Catatonia	22
Fecal incontinence (smearing)	13

Table 1.1 Manic episodes: mean rate of symptom occurrence. Adapted from Goodwin and Jamison [4].

Depression

The term 'depression' is commonly applied to non-clinical emotional states as well as being used to designate a range of dysphoric states, including those meeting criteria for MDEs. Patients with MDEs are characterized by a loss of ability to experience pleasure in activities that are usually fun or exciting, rather than the degree to which they feel sad. The DSM-IV-TR criteria for MDEs require the presence of five symptoms – including depressed mood or decreased interest – for most of the day nearly every day for a period of 2 weeks or longer.

The course of bipolar disorder generally includes both major and minor depressive episodes and symptoms. There is little agreement on the differences between unipolar and bipolar types of depression. Potter proposed some possible distinguishing factors (Table 1.2) [6], and in a follow-up study of 'pseudo-unipolar depression', Maj et al found some differences (Table 1.3) [7]. Somatic and anxiety residual symptoms may

Clinical differences between bipolar and unipolar depression	
Bipolar depression	**Unipolar depression**
Calm withdrawal	More physical and mental activity
Psychomotor retardation	Somatic complaints
Hypersomnia	Sleep disorder
Fewer anxiety symptoms, less somatic complaints	Anxiety
Less anger	Anger

Table 1.2 Clinical differences between bipolar and unipolar depression. Generally, the bipolar patient is less conscious of and complains less of depression and dysphoria. There is a greater risk for this type of patient not to be treated and for them to commit suicide. Adapted with permission from Potter [6].

Variables significantly associated with bipolar outcome in patients with major depression		
Variable	**Sensitivity (%)**	**Specificity (%)**
Pharmacological hypomania	32	100
Bipolar family history	56	98
Loaded pedigrees	32	95
Hypersomnic, retarded depression	59	88
Psychotic depression	42	85
Postpartum onset	58	84
Onset of depression before age 26 years	71	68

Table 1.3 Variables significantly associated with bipolar outcome in patients with major depression. Adapted with permission from Maj et al [7].

be more common in unipolar depression [8], whereas atypical features may be more prevalent in bipolar depression, and particularly in bipolar II depression [9]. As a cross-sectional differentiation between unipolar and bipolar depression does not appear to be possible [10], the International Society for Bipolar Disorders Task Force has proposed a probabilistic approach to the diagnosis of bipolar depression [11,12].

Subclinical depressive symptoms can linger even in those who have clinically stabilised bipolar disorder. A 16-week cohort study found subclinical depression in nearly 17% of clinically stable patients. Rates of depressive symptoms were similar between the bipolar I and bipolar II groups, and were highest in patients with rapid cycling [13].

Mixed

Mixed episodes are characterized by the presence of manic symptoms as well as depressive symptoms, with a duration of at least 1 week. Because both manic and depressive features must meet the full diagnostic criteria, mixed episodes are difficult to diagnose. More frequent are dysphoric manic episodes (or depressive and/or anxious mania) presenting with at least two typical depressive symptoms. Other types of mixed states, such as agitated depressions, have been poorly studied [14].

A recent study of 134 patients with bipolar I disorder found that 34.3% had a history of pure manic episodes (PMA), 26.1% had a history of pure mixed episodes (PMIX), and 39.5% had a history of both manic and mixed episodes (MIX). Significantly higher rates of depressive predominant polarity, Axis I comorbidity, and suicidal ideation were noted in the PMIX group [15].

Epidemiology
Lifetime prevalence

Epidemiological evidence suggests that the lifetime prevalence of strictly defined bipolar I disorder in the western population is around 1% (range: 0.5–1.6%) [16,17]. This rate is consistent across diverse cultures and ethnic groups [18]. The epidemiology of bipolar II disorder is less well established but, using a conservative definition, it is believed to have a lifetime prevalence of around 1.5–2.5% [19,20]. Whereas bipolar I disorder affects men and women fairly equally, bipolar II is more common in women [20,21]. Men are also more likely to present with any predominant polarity [21].

For the full spectrum of bipolar illness, including subthreshold mania and depression, estimates of the lifetime prevalence range from 4% to 12% [22]. The National Comorbidity Survey replication study found a lifetime prevalence of bipolar disorders in the US amongst adults and adolescents to be 4.8% (0.6% bipolar I; 1.8% bipolar II; 2.4% subthreshold bipolar) [23,24]. The wide variability reflects differences in diagnostic criteria as well as the unreliability of the initial diagnosis. Some groups, such as young patients with psychotic depression, are especially likely to be misdiagnosed: as many as 50% of patients hospitalized with unipolar depression are eventually diagnosed with bipolar disorder (Figure 1.1) [25].

The BRIDGE study was a multinational, cross-sectional trial designed to determine the frequency of bipolar symptoms in patients in treatment for a current MDE. Of the 5635 patients surveyed, 16.1% fulfilled the DSM-IV-TR criteria for bipolar disorder. This expanded to 47% when the bipolar specificity criteria were applied [26].

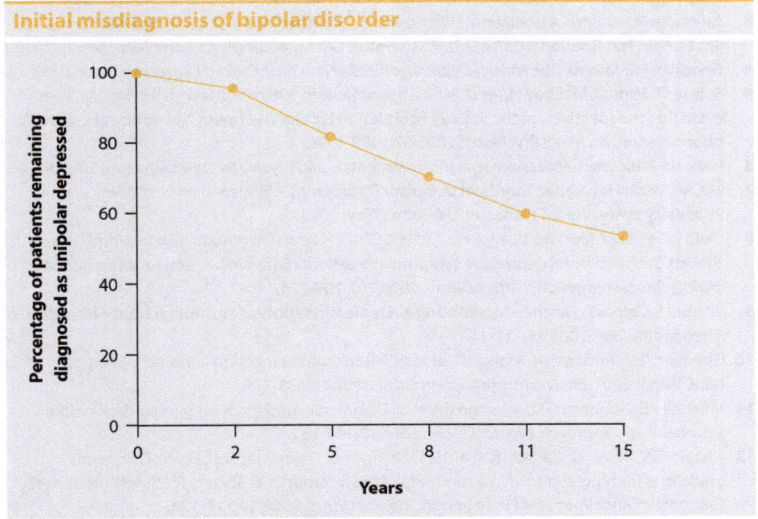

Figure 1.1 Initial misdiagnosis of bipolar disorder. Data taken from Goldberg et al [25].

Age of onset

The first episode of bipolar disorder typically occurs in the second or third decade of life, with the peak age of onset between 15 and 25 years. However, there is often an interval of 5–10 years between the age at onset and first treatment or first hospitalization [27].

Onset of mania before the age of 15 has been less well studied, and diagnosing bipolar disorder in this age group may be complicated by its atypical presentation with attention deficit hyperactivity disorder. Thus, the true age at onset of bipolar disorder is still unclear and may be younger than reported for the full syndrome [28].

Onset of mania in individuals over 60 years of age is less likely to have a genetic basis; rather, it tends to be associated with underlying organic illness such as stroke or central nervous system lesions [29].

The particular diagnostic challenges presented by these patient subgroups are discussed further in Chapter 4.

References

1   World Health Organization. *The ICD-10 Classification of Mental and Behavioral Disorders: Clinical Description and Diagnostic Guidelines (CDDG-10)*. Geneva: WHO; 1992.
2   World Health Organization. *The ICD-10 Classification of Mental and Behavioral Disorders: Diagnostic Criteria for Research (DCR-10)*. Geneva: WHO; 1993.
3   American Psychiatric Association. *Diagnostic and Statistical Manual of Mental Disorders, 4th Edition, Text Revision (DSM-IV-TR)*. Washington DC: American Psychiatric Association; 2000.
4   Goodwin FK, Jamison KR. *Manic–Depressive Illness*. New York: Oxford University Press; 1990.
5   Suppes T, Mintz J, McElroy SL, et al. Mixed hypomania in 908 patients with bipolar disorder evaluated prospectively in the Stanley Foundation Bipolar Treatment Network: a sex-specific phenomenon. *Arch Gen Psychiatry*. 2005;62:1089-1096.
6   Potter WZ. Bipolar depression: specific treatments. *J Clin Psychiatry*. 1998;59(suppl 18):30-36.
7   Maj M, Akiskal HS, Lopez-Ibor JJ, et al. *Bipolar Disorder*. WPA Evidence and Experience in Psychiatry series, Vol 5. Chichester, UK: John Wiley; 2002.
8   Vieta E, Sánchez-Moreno J, Lahuerta J, et al; EDHIPO Group (Hypomania Detection Study Group). Subsyndromal depressive symptoms in patients with bipolar and unipolar disorder during clinical remission. *J Affect Disord*. 2008;107:169-174.
9   Brugue E, Colom F, Sanchez-Moreno J, et al. Depression subtypes in bipolar I and II disorders. *Psychopathology*. 2008;41:111-114.
10 Goodwin GM, Anderson I, Arango C, et al. ECNP consensus meeting. Bipolar depression. Nice, March 2007. *Eur Neuropsychopharmacol*. 2008;18:535-549.
11 Mitchell PB, Goodwin GM, Johnson GF, et al. Diagnostic guidelines for bipolar depression: a probabilistic approach. *Bipolar Disord*. 2008;10:144-152.
12 Ghaemi SN, Bauer M, Cassidy F, et al; ISBD Diagnostic Guidelines Task Force. Diagnostic guidelines for bipolar disorder: a summary of the International Society for Bipolar Disorders Diagnostic Guidelines Task Force Report. *Bipolar Disord*. 2008;10:117-128.

13 Vieta E, de Arce R, Jiménez-Arriero MA, et al. Detection of subclinical depression in bipolar disorder: a cross-sectional, 4-month prospective follow-up study at community mental health services (SIN-DEPRES). *J Clin Psychiatry*. 2010;71:1465-1474.

14 Vieta E. Bipolar mixed states and their treatment. *Expert Rev Neurother*. 2005;5:63-68.

15 Pacchiarotti I, Mazzarini L, Kotzalidis GD, et al. Mania and depression. Mixed, not stirred. *J Affect Disord*. 2011;133:105-113.

16 Kessler RC, Berglund P, Demler O, et al. Lifetime prevalence and age-of-onset distributions of DSM-IV disorders in the National Comorbidity Survey Replication. *Arch Gen Psychiatry*. 2005;62:593-602.

17 Hirschfeld RM, Calabrese JR, Weissman MM, et al. Screening for bipolar disorder in the community. *J Clin Psychiatry*. 2003;64:53-59.

18 Merikangas KR, Jin R, He J-P, et al. Prevalence and correlates of bipolar spectrum disorder in the World Mental Health Survey Initiative. *Arch Gen Psychiatry*. 2011;68:241-251.

19 Amsterdam JD, Brunswick DJ. Antidepressant monotherapy for bipolar type II major depression. *Bipolar Disord*. 2003;5:388-395.

20 Hantouche EG, Adiskal HS, Lancrenon S, et al. Systematic clinical methodology for validating bipolar-II disorder: data in mid-stream from a French national multi-site study (EPIDEP). *J Affect Disord*. 1998;50:163-173.

21 Nivoli AMA, Pacchiarotti I, Rosa AR, et al. Gender differences in a cohort study of 604 patients: the role of predominant polarity. *J Affect Disord*. 2011;133:443-449.

22 Angst J. Gamma A, Benazzi F, et al. Toward a re-definition of subthreshold bipolarity: epidemiology and proposed criteria for bipolar-II, minor bipolar disorders and hypomania. *J Affect Disord*. 2003; 73:133-146.

23 Merikangas KR, Akiskal HS, Angst J, et al. Lifetime and 12-month prevalence of bipolar spectrum disorder in the National Comorbidity Survey replication. *Arch Gen Psychiatry*. 2007;64:543-552.

24 Kessler RC, Petukhova M, Sampson NA, et al. Twelve-month and lifetime prevalence and lifetime morbid risk of anxiety and mood disorders in the United States. *Int J Methods Psychiatr Res*. 2012;21:169-184.

25 Goldberg JF, Harrow M, Whiteside JE. Risk for bipolar Illness in patients initially hospitalized for unipolar depression. Am J Psychiatry 2001; 158:1265-1270.

26 Angst J, Azorin JM, Bowden CH, et al; the BRIDGE Study Group. Prevalence and characteristics of undiagnosed bipolar disorders in patients with a major depressive episode: the BRIDGE Study. *Arch Gen Psychiatry*. 2011;68:791-799.

27 Lish JD, Dime-Meenan S, Whybrow PC, et al. The National Depressive and Manic-Depressive Association (DMDA) survey of bipolar members. *J Affect Disord*. 1994;31:281-294.

28 Hirschfeld RMA, Bowden CL, Perlis RH, et al. American Psychiatric Association. Practice guideline for the treatment of patients with bipolar disorder [Revision]. *Am J Psychiatry*. 2002;159(4 suppl):1-50.

29 McDonald WM, Nemeroff CB. The diagnosis and treatment of mania in the elderly. *Bull Menninger Clin*. 1996;60:174-196.

Chapter 2

Psychosocial consequences

Quality of life
Personal burden

Bipolar disorder has significant psychosocial consequences for the patient, and may have a devastating impact on personal, occupational, and family life [1]. The first episode of bipolar illness typically occurs between 17 and 21 years of age, a time associated with education, career, and social development [2]. Those with bipolar disorder are two to three times more likely to be divorced and their occupational status is twice as likely to deteriorate versus non-bipolar individuals [3]. In recognition of these negative consequences, the World Health Organization (WHO) has identified bipolar disorder as the twelfth leading cause of disability worldwide [4].

Even with optimal treatment, people with bipolar disorder spend around half their time with symptoms [5]. Episodes of depression are associated with greater impairment in work, family, and social life than episodes of mania (Figure 2.1) [6]. After remission of an acute episode, many patients do not fully recover their ability to function in work and social activities, and the presence of subsyndromal depressive symptoms is strongly associated with functional disability [7,8]. While one study found a significant improvement in global functioning 6 months after an acute episode or subsyndromal state, only 26% of patients achieved favorable function, even with continuous therapy [9].

E. Vieta, *Managing Bipolar Disorder in Clinical Practice*, DOI: 10.1007/978-1-908517-94-4_2, © Springer Healthcare 2013

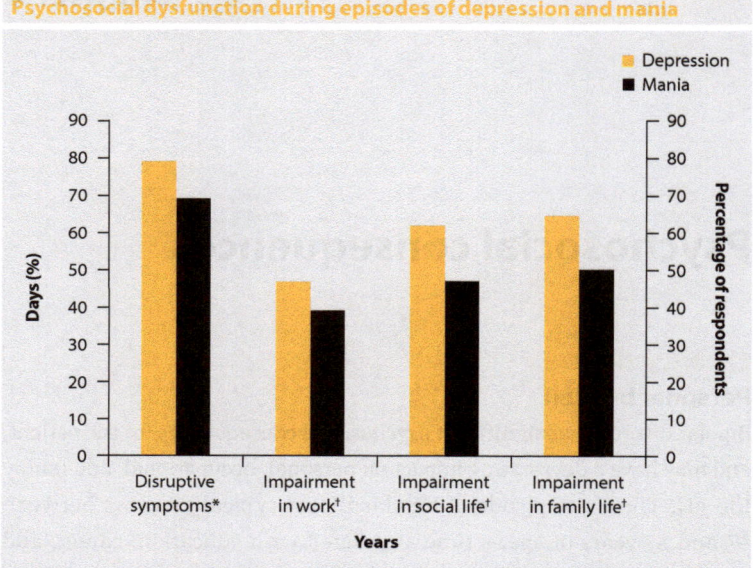

Figure 2.1 Psychosocial dysfunction during episodes of depression and mania. *Within 12 months before survey; †Within 4 weeks before survey. Reproduced from Post [6].

Patients who have had multiple episodes often have worse psychosocial functioning than first-episode patients. A one-year follow-up outcome study noted that patients at first episode had better functioning, including lower cognitive impairment and higher autonomy levels. Fewer patients with multiple episodes had symptomatic recovery [10].

Compared with healthy individuals, people with bipolar disorder report significantly less satisfaction with their quality of life. A community survey found that individuals who screened positive for bipolar disorder using the Mood Disorder Questionnaire experienced many more difficulties with work-related performance, leisure activities, and social and family interactions than those who screened negative. They were also more likely to have been arrested, convicted, or jailed for a crime [5].

Bipolar patients in remission are often still seriously disabled in their occupational functioning, interpersonal relationships, cognitive performance, autonomy, and finances [11]. Other studies have also shown that patients with bipolar disorder can be rated similarly in terms of health-related quality of life (HRQoL) to individuals with unipolar depression (major depressive disorder) but equal to if not lower than those with chronic medical illnesses [12]. Furthermore, improvements in HRQoL scores take longer to be seen than symptomatic improvement [13] and there is evidence that, with recurrent bipolar episodes, progressive deterioration in functioning may occur [14,15].

In the EMBLEM study, just 11% of over 3500 manic patients reported no work impairment during the year before the manic episode [16]. In the same study, a significant number of patients still had high work impairment even after 2 years of maintenance therapy. Factors associated with higher work impairment included lower education levels, high impairment at baseline, and rapid cycling [17].

Another study of primary care patients found that those who screened positive for bipolar disorder suffered significant disability in health, social, family, and occupational functioning [18]. In this study, impaired HRQoL remained significantly associated with a positive screen for bipolar disorder, even after adjusting for the presence of any current mental condition. Moreover, nearly one-fifth of those who screened positive for bipolar disorder reported suicidal ideation in the previous 2 weeks, compared with just 4% of those who screened negative. Suicide risk is discussed in more detail in Chapter 5.

Patients who were hospitalized for bipolar depression early in the course of illness were followed up 6 months later to determine occupational and social adjustment. Even after 6 months, occupational recovery and social adjustment were limited, and a majority of patients still had mood symptoms [19].

Economic burden

Bipolar disorder also greatly increases healthcare utilization and the need for welfare and disability benefits. Indeed, people with bipolar disorder have been shown to use more healthcare services than people with depression or chronic medical illnesses [12].

In the US, the direct costs of bipolar disorder were estimated at US$30.7 billion in 2009 [20]. Much of this amount is attributed to inpatient care: in one study, the overall rate of hospital admission among individuals with bipolar illness was 39%, whereas the rate of admission specifically for bipolar disorder was 13% [20]. Other direct costs include outpatient medical care, as well as non-treatment-related expenditures (eg, use of the criminal justice system). In the same year, indirect costs (primarily related to lost productivity of wage-earners, homemakers, persons in institutions, and those who committed suicide) were estimated at over US$120.3 billion [21]. The most extensive study in Europe [21], including both direct and indirect costs, estimated UK national costs of bipolar disorder at £342 billion (about €431.5 million). In this study, the costs associated with hospitalization of patients during acute episodes appear to represent the largest share of direct costs, at £206 million per year [22].

Comorbidity
Psychiatric comorbidity
Bipolar disorder is associated with a high rate of psychiatric comorbidity. Indeed, it is uncommon to find a patient with bipolar disorder who does not meet criteria for at least one other DSM-IV-TR disorder: in the US National Comorbidity Survey, the prevalence of axis I disorders among patients with bipolar I was 100% [23]. Axis I disorders have also been noted in patients with bipolar II [24].

The most frequent psychiatric comorbidities are anxiety disorders, alcohol and substance abuse, and attention deficit hyperactivity disorder (ADHD), all of which greatly increase a patient's overall psychosocial vulnerability. Both axis I and axis II comorbid conditions have been shown to be associated with an earlier age at onset and a worse course of bipolar illness [6,25].

The relationship between psychiatric comorbid conditions and bipolar disorder is likely to be bidirectional. Successful treatment of bipolar disorder often improves comorbidities and vice versa. There are some exceptions, however. Antidepressant medications to treat obsessive–compulsive disorder and stimulants to treat ADHD often exacerbate symptoms of bipolar disorder and may precipitate a manic episode [26].

Individuals with bipolar disorder frequently exhibit alcohol or substance abuse, which may magnify the severity of illness and increase the likelihood of hospitalization. Women with bipolar disorder are more than seven times as likely to suffer from alcohol dependency compared with the general population. In men with bipolar disorder, the risk of alcoholism is increased nearly threefold [27]. Abuse of illicit drugs, particularly stimulants, is more relevant to younger patients with mania and again is associated with worse outcomes. However, there is evidence that effective treatment of substance misuse can improve compliance and bipolar disorder outcomes [28].

The association between bipolar disorder and eating disorders has been documented in several epidemiological studies [24,29–31]. Interestingly, anywhere from 6% to 15% of bipolar disorder patients may have eating disorders, and the lifetime prevalence of bipolar disorder among individuals with anorexia or bulimia is about 8%, which is greater than what is seen in the general population [32]. Seasonal variations in food intake, including carbohydrate craving during winter depressions, are common in bipolar II disorder, and affect women four times as often as men [33]. Binge eating is also common, being reported by as many as 38% of bipolar patients in one study [34]. The prevalence of subthreshold eating disorders may be even higher [35].

Non-psychiatric comorbidity

Bipolar disorder is associated with both obesity (21–32% of patients) and being overweight (58%) [36–39]. The causes include not only eating disorders, but also inactivity, lithium-related subclinical hypothyroidism, and weight gain as a side effect of some antipsychotic drugs [40,41]. Another drug-related side effect, dry mouth, can also lead to weight gain through increased consumption of high-calorie drinks. Obesity, in turn, is associated with a myriad of complications, such as diabetes and cardiovascular disease, which diminish a patient's quality of life and reduce longevity. Obesity has been shown to be a significant correlate of poor outcomes in patients with bipolar I disorder [42].

Bipolar disorder is associated with a range of other non-psychiatric comorbidities. The findings are summarized in Tables 2.1 and 2.2 [43]. In a relatively young series of bipolar patients (mean age 32.8 years), 13.6% had endocrine and metabolic diseases, including diabetes, obesity,

Comorbid medical conditions in 1379 outpatients with bipolar I disorder		
Comorbidity	**Number of patients**	**Percentage**
Infectious and parasitic diseases	105	7.6
Neoplasms	39	2.8
Endocrine, nutritional, and metabolic disease	187	13.6
Diseases of blood	21	1.5
Diseases of the nervous system and sense organs	147	10.7
Diseases of the circulatory system	179	13.0
Diseases of the respiratory system	101	7.3
Diseases of the digestive system	101	7.3
Diseases of the genitourinary system	51	3.7
Complications of pregnancy, childbirth, and the puerperium	5	0.4
Diseases of the skin and subcutaneous tissues	28	2.0
Diseases of the musculoskeletal system and injury	141	10.7
Other	13	0.9

Table 2.1 Comorbid medical conditions in 1379 outpatients with bipolar I disorder.
Reproduced with permission from Beyer et al [43].

Specific illnesses in 1379 outpatients with bipolar I disorder		
Disorder	**Number of patients**	**Percent (%)**
Cardiac disease/hypertension	146	10.7
COPD/asthma	84	6.1
Diabetes	59	4.3
HIV	39	2.8
Hepatitis C	26	1.9

Table 2.2 Specific illnesses in 1379 outpatients with bipolar I disorder. COPD, chronic obstructive pulmonary disease. Reproduced with permission from Beyer et al [43].

thyroid diseases, and hypercholesterolemia, 13.0% suffered from diseases of the circulatory system, including heart disease and hypertension, and 10.7% had diseases of the nervous system or sense organs [43]. The global prevalence rates of metabolic syndrome in bipolar patients have been found to range from 16.7% to as high as 54% [44]. Patients with bipolar disorder and metabolic syndrome have more complex illness, more frequent suicide attempts, and a lower likelihood of recovery [45].

The need for early intervention

Given the negative consequences of bipolar disorder for the patient as well as for their family, friends, and wider society, there is clearly a place for effective management strategies. With adequate containment of their disease, patients with bipolar disorder can improve their social and occupational functioning, sustain high work productivity, and achieve acceptable HRQoL, which in turn should reduce service utilization and lifetime healthcare costs. Moreover, effective treatment may reduce the high morbidity and mortality (including suicide) associated with bipolar disorder.

An interesting feature of early intervention is the potential to modify the underlying disease course. As noted previously, there is evidence that patients' functional status deteriorates progressively with recurrent episodes of bipolar illness. A study of patients with bipolar disorder found that, compared with multiple-episode mania, those experiencing first-episode mania had a significantly shorter duration of hospitalization and a higher rate of comorbid impulse control disorders [15].

This finding supports the kindling or sensitization model, which posits that regular and frequent periods of nervous system activation (such as affective episodes) may predispose individuals to additional recurrences in an accelerated and automatic fashion. Similar to recurrent episodes in epilepsy, initial bipolar mood episodes tend to arise in connection with interpersonal, chronobiological, or environmental factors, whereas later episodes, once 'kindled', may occur spontaneously and independently of external triggers [46]. Neurobiological mechanisms that have been suggested to underlie recurrent episodes include second messenger systems and gene transcription and/or translation [47].

Although empirical studies have not validated a kindling mechanism to explain bipolar disorder recurrence, there are substantial clinical data to support a relationship between relapse and episode regularity or periodicity. In a longitudinal study of patients with bipolar disorder, remission at two or more follow-up visits was associated with remission at 10-year follow-up, leading the authors to suggest that early and sustained remission is related to better subsequent psychosocial functioning and continued remission [48].

Whether or not successive bipolar episodes lead to progressive neurodegenerative changes remains the subject of debate. Deterioration in clinical and functional status may be the consequence of a neurobiological process [49]; conversely, the adverse psychosocial consequences of illness chronicity could produce clinical deterioration independently of a primary neurodegenerative process [50].

Evidence for progressive neurodegeneration includes the presence of persistent cognitive deficits during periods of euthymia [14], as well as the fact that bipolar disorder patients with enduring cognitive deficits tend to be older and have a more chronic illness course and multiple episodes [51]. However, abnormalities in amygdala volume appear similar in pediatric and adult bipolar disorder patients [52], and between first-episode and multiple-episode patients [53], suggesting that not all functional neuroanatomical deficits in bipolar disorder necessarily reflect a progressive degeneration. Although a subgroup of bipolar patients may show cognitive impairment primarily related to mutations in some genes involved in neuronal migration and neurodevelopment [54], the majority may respond better to a model of neurodegeneration [55], in which cognitive impairment, medical comorbidities, and poor functional outcome may correlate with the number of episodes and biological changes related to the concept of allostatic load [56]. This model would provide a strong rationale for early intervention [49,57] and rehabilitation [58].

References

1   Reinares M, Vieta E, Colom F, et al. What really matters to bipolar patients' caregivers: sources of family burden. *J Affect Disord*. 2006;94:157-163.
2   Carter TD, Mundo E, Parikh SV, et al. Early age at onset as a risk factor for poor outcome of bipolar disorder. *J Psychiatr Res*. 2003;37:297-303.
3   Manning JS, Haykal RF, Connor PD, et al. On the nature of depressive and anxious states in a family practice setting: the high prevalence of bipolar II and related disorders in a cohort followed longitudinally. *Compr Psychiatry*. 1997;38:102-108.
4   World Health Organization (WHO). The global burden of disease. 2004 update. WHO website. www.who.int/entity/healthinfo/global_burden_disease/GBD_report_2004update_full.pdf. Accessed September 17, 2012.
5   Calabrese J, Hirschfeld R, Reed M, et al. Impact of bipolar disorder on a US community sample. *J Clin Psychiatry*. 2003;64:425-432.
6   Post RM. The impact of bipolar depression. *J Clin Psychiatry*. 2005;66(suppl 5):5-10.
7   Montoya A, Tohen M, Vieta E, et al. Functioning and symptomatic outcomes in patients with bipolar I disorder in syndromal remission: a 1-year, prospective, observational cohort study. *J Affect Disord*. 2010;127:50-57.

8   Bonnín CM, Sánchez-Moreno J, Martínez-Arán A, et al. Subthreshold symptoms in bipolar disorder: impact on neurocognition, quality of life and disability. *J Affect Disord.* 2012;13:650-659.

9   Rosa AR, Reinares M, Amman B, et al. Six-month functional outcome of a bipolar disorder cohort in the context of a specialized-case program. *Bipolar Disord.* 2011;13:679-686.

10 Rosa AR, González-Ortega I, González-Pinto A, et al. One-year psychosocial functioning in patients in the early vs. late stage of bipolar disorder. *Acta Psychiatr Scand.* 2012;125:335-341.

11 Rosa AR, Franco C, Martinez-Aran A, et al. Functional impairment in patients with remitted bipolar disorder. *Psychotherapy Psychosom.* 2008;77:390-392.

12 Dean BB, Gerner D, Gerner RH. A systematic review evaluating health-related quality of life, work impairment, and healthcare costs and utilization in bipolar disorder. *Curr Med Res Opin.* 2004;20:139-154.

13 Dion GL, Tohen M, Anthony WA, et al. Symptoms and functioning of patients with bipolar disorder six months after hospitalization. *Hosp Community Psychiatry.* 1988; 39:652-657.

14 Martinez-Arán A, Vieta E, Colom F, et al. Cognitive impairment in euthymic bipolar patients: implications for clinical and functional outcome. *Bipolar Disord.* 2004;6:224-232.

15 Keck PE, McElroy SL, Strakowski SM, et al. Outcome and comorbidity in first-episode compared with multiple-episode mania. *J Nerv Ment Dis.* 1995;183:320-324.

16 Goetz I, Tohen M, Reed C, et al. Functional impairment in patients with mania: baseline results from the EMBLEM study. *Bipolar Disord.* 2006;9:45-52.

17 Reed C, Goetz I, Vieta E, et al; the EMBLEM Advisory Board. Work impairment in bipolar disorder–results from a two-year observational study (EMBLEM). *Eur Psychiatry.* 2010;25:338-344.

18 Das AK, Olfson M, Gameroff MJ, et al. Screening for bipolar disorder in a primary care practice. JAMA 2005; 293:956-963.

19 Dickerson F, Origoni A, Stallings C, et al. Occupational status and social adjustment six months after hospitalization early in the course of bipolar disorder: a prospective study. *Bipolar Disord.* 2010;12:10-20.

20 Peele PB, Xu Y, Kupfer DJ. Insurance expenditures on bipolar disorder: clinical and parity implications. *Am J Psychiatry.* 2003;160:1286-1290.

21 Dilsaver SC. An estimate of the minimum economic burden of bipolar I and II disorders in the United States: 2009. *J Affect Disord.* 2011;129:79-83.

22 Young AH, Rigney U, Shaw S, et al. Annual cost of managing bipolar disorder to the UK healthcare system. *J Affect Disord.* 2011;133:450-456.

23 Kessler RC, Stang P, Wittchen HU, et al. Lifetime co-morbidities between social phobia and mood disorders in the US National Comorbidity Survey. *Psychol Med.* 1999;29:555-567.

24 Mantere O, Isometsä E, Ketokivi M, et al. A prospective latent analyses study of psychiatric comorbidity of DSM-IV bipolar I and II disorders. *Bipolar Disord.* 2010;12:271-284.

25 McElroy S, Altshuler L, Suppes T, et al. Axis I psychiatric comorbidity and its relationship to historical illness variables in 288 patients with bipolar disorder. *Am J Psychiatry.* 2001;158:420-426.

26 Skirrow C, Hosang GM, Farmer AE, et al. An update on the debated association between ADHD and bipolar disorder across the lifespan. *J Affect Disord.* 2012;141:143-159.

27 Frye MA, Altshuler LL, McElroy SL et al. Gender differences in prevalence, risk, and clinical correlates of alcoholism comorbidity in bipolar disorder. *Am J Psychiatry.* 2003;160:883-889.

28 Salloum IM, Thase ME. Impact of substance abuse on the course and treatment of bipolar disorder. *Bipolar Disord.* 2000;2:269-280.

29 Kaye W, Weltzin TE, Hsu LKG, et al. Patients with anorexia nervosa have elevated scores on Yale-Brown Obsessive Scale. *Int J Eat Disord.* 1992;12:57-62.

30 Simpson SG, al-Mufti R, Andersen AE et al. Bipolar II affective disorder in eating disorder inpatients. *J Nerv Ment Dis.* 1992;180:719-722.

31 Vieta E, Colom F, Martínez-Arán A, et al. Bipolar II disorder and comorbidity. *Compr Psychiatry*. 2000;41:339-343.

32 McElroy SL, Kotwal R, Keck PE Jr. Comorbidity of eating disorders with bipolar disorder and treatment implications. *Bipolar Disord*. 2006;8:686-695.

33 Wehr TA, Rosenthal NE. Seasonality and affective illness. *Am J Psychiatry*. 1989;146:829-839.

34 Kruger S, Shugar G, Cooke RG. Comorbidity of binge eating disorder and the partial binge eating syndrome with bipolar disorder. *Int J Eat Disord*. 1996;19:45-52.

35 Torrent C, Vieta E, Garcia-Garcia M; Spanish Working Group for the Validation of the Barcelona Bipolar Eating Disorder Scale (BEDS). Validation of the Barcelona Bipolar Eating Disorder Scale for bipolar patients with eating disturbances. *Psychopathology*. 2008;41:379-387.

36 Elmslie JL, Silverstone JT, Mann JI, et al. Prevalence of overweight and obesity in bipolar patients. *J Clin Psychiatry*. 2000;61:179-184.

37 Elmslie JL, Mann JI, Silverstone JT, et al. Determinants of overweight and obesity in patients with bipolar disorder. *J Clin Psychiatry*. 2001; 62:486-491.

38 Fagiolini A, Frank E, Houck MSH, et al. Prevalence of obesity and weight change during the treatment in patients with bipolar I disorder. *J Clin Psychiatry*. 2002;63:528-533.

39 McElroy SL, Frye MA, Suppes T, et al. Correlates of overweight and obesity in 644 patients with bipolar disorder. *J Clin Psychiatry*. 2002;63:207-213.

40 Allison DB, Casey DE. Antipsychotic-induced weight gain: a review of the literature. *J Clin Psychiatry*. 2001;62(suppl 7):22-31.

41 Chengappa KN, Chalassani L, Brar JS, et al. Changes in body weight and body mass index among psychiatric patients receiving lithium, valproate, or topiramate: an open-label, nonrandomized chart review. *Clin Ther*. 2002;24:1576-1584.

42 Fagiolini A, Kupfer DJ, Houck PR, et al. Obesity as a correlate of outcome in patients with bipolar I disorder. *Am J Psychiatry*. 2003;160:112-117.

43 Beyer J, Kuchibhatla M, Gersing K, et al. Medical comorbidity in a bipolar outpatient clinical population. *Neuropsychopharmacol*. 2005;30:401-404.

44 de Almeida KM, Moreira CLRL, Lafer B. Metabolic syndrome and bipolar disorder: what should psychiatrists know? *CNS Neurosci Ther*. 2012;18:160-166.

45 McIntyre RS, Alsuwaidan M, Goldstein BI, et al. The Canadian Network for Mood and Anxiety Treatments (CANMAT) task force recommendations for the management of patients with mood disorders and comorbid metabolic disorders. *Ann Clin Psychiatry*. 2012;24:69-84.

46 Post RM, Rubinow DR, Ballenger JC. Conditioning and sensitization in the longitudinal course of affective illness. *Br J Psychiatry*. 1986;149:191-201.

47 Ghaemi SN, Boiman EE, Goodwin FK. Kindling and second messengers: An approach to the neurobiology of recurrence in bipolar disorder. *Biol Psychiatry*. 1999;45:137-144.

48 Goldberg JF, Harrow M. Consistency of remission and outcome in bipolar and unipolar mood disorders:a 10-year prospective follow-up. *J Affect Disord*. 2004;81:123-131.

49 Berk M, Conus P, Kapczinski F, et al. From neuroprogression to neuroprotection: implications for clinical care. *Med J Aust*. 2010;193(4 suppl):S36-S40.

50 Goldberg JF, Garno JL, Harrow M. Long-term remission and recovery in bipolar disorder: a review. *Curr Psychiatry Rep*. 2005;7:456-461.

51 Bearden CE, Hoffman KM, Cannon TD. The neuropsychology and neuroanatomy of bipolar disorder: a critical review. *Bipolar Disord*. 2001;3:106-150.

52 Blumberg HP, Kaufman J, Martin A, et al. Amygdala and hippocampal volumes in adolescents and adults with bipolar disorder. *Arch Gen Psychiatry*. 2003; 60:1201-1218.

53 Strakowski SM, DelBello MP, Sax KW, et al. Brain magnetic resonance imaging of structural abnormalities in bipolar disorder. *Arch Gen Psychiatry*. 1999; 56:254-260.

54 Tabares-Seisdedos R, Escamez T, Martinez-Gimenez JA, et al. Variations in genes regulating neuronal migration predict reduced prefrontal cognition in schizophrenia and bipolar subjects from mediterranean Spain: A preliminary study. *Neuroscience*. 2006;139:1289-1300.

55 Goodwin GM, Martinez-Aran A, Glahn DC, et al. Cognitive Impairment in Bipolar Disorder: Neurodevelopment or Neurodegeneration? An ECNP expert meeting report. *Eur Neuropsychopharmacol*. 2008;18:787-793.

56 Kapczinski F, Vieta E, Andreazza AC, et al. Allostatic load in bipolar disorder: implications for pathophysiology and treatment. *Neurosci Biobehav Rev*. 2008;32:675-692.

57 Vieta E, Reinares M, Rosa AR. Staging bipolar disorder. *Neurotox Res*. 2011;19:279-285.

58 Vieta E, Rosa AR. Evolving trends in the long-term treatment of bipolar disorder. *World J Biol Psychiatry*. 2007;8:4-11.

Chapter 3

Etiology and disease course

Etiology
Biological factors

Epidemiological and genetic evidence suggest that bipolar disorder has a strong hereditary component and that prevalence is relatively insensitive to variations in personal or social adversity [1]. First-degree relatives of patients with bipolar disorder have significantly higher rates of mood disorders (including bipolar I, bipolar II, and major depressive disorder) than relatives of non-psychiatrically ill comparison groups [2].

Nevertheless, bipolar disorder does not have a simple mendelian pattern of inheritance; rather, it is presumed that many genes with small interacting effects contribute to the clinical syndrome. Based on information from twin studies, the heritability of bipolar disorder has been estimated at 79% [3].

Multiple linkage loci and candidate genes have been identified in molecular genetic studies of bipolar disorder. In particular, there is evidence of associated genetic polymorphisms in the expression of genes encoding transporters and receptors of biogenic amines [4,5]. However, none of these findings has been consistently replicated [6], and meta-analyses have also reported conflicting results [7]. A meta-analysis of existing candidate gene studies identified the following regions which are associated with susceptibility to bipolar disorder [8]:

- 1p36.22;
- 3q13.31 & q13.33;
- 5p15.333;

E. Vieta, *Managing Bipolar Disorder in Clinical Practice*,
DOI: 10.1007/978-1-908517-94-4_3, © Springer Healthcare 2013

- 6p21.3;
- 11p14.1 & p15.5;
- 11q23.1–q23.2;
- 12p13.31;
- 13q14.2 & q-33.2;
- 17q11.2 & q23.2;
- 22q11.21;
- Xp11.3; and
- Xq23.

Interestingly, several overlap with regions implicated in schizophrenia [9]. A study designed to assess the genetic overlap between schizophrenia and bipolar disorder found a substantial link between the conditions. First-degree relatives of patients with schizophrenia were at increased risk to develop bipolar disorder and vice versa [10]. The rs27072 single nucleotide polymorphism in the dopamine transporter gene has also been associated with bipolar disorder [11].

A number of other biological mechanisms have been postulated in the etiology of bipolar disorder. These include hypothalamic–pituitary–adrenal axis abnormalities, thyroid abnormalities, neurotransmitter/receptor imbalances (especially involving dopaminergic activity), second messenger abnormalities, and mitochondrial dysfunction [12]. Insights from recent imaging studies are discussed in more detail in a later section.

Environmental factors

Environmental factors must play a role in the development of bipolar disorder, since identical twins are frequently discordant for the condition [3,9,13]. Indeed, a growing body of evidence suggests that environmental factors have an important impact on the onset, course, and expression of bipolar disorder.

Numerous studies have shown that recent negative and/or stressful life events predict the likelihood of onset and recurrence of mood episodes [14]. The BRIDGE trial noted that women who had a first episode of postpartum depression had a greater prevalence of bipolar disorder than women whose first episode of depression was not postpartum-related [15]. Moreover, most studies have found that negative life events precede manic/hypomanic as well as depressive episodes. Sleep deprivation and disruption of daily social rhythms (eg, meal times, sleep–wake times) have been implicated as a final common pathway in this relationship [16]. Even sunlight has been found to play a role in the development of bipolar disorder. In a global study of 2414 patients, the larger the maximum monthly increase in solar insulation during springtime the younger the age of disease onset [17].

The presence of supportive or non-supportive interpersonal relationships is also known to influence the course of bipolar disorder. It is thought that social support from family or friends can 'buffer' against the deleterious effects of stress or directly enhance functioning among bipolar individuals, whereas criticism and emotional over-involvement (high 'expressed emotion') can cause additional stress and worsen the disease course [14].

There is growing interest in the role of cognition in bipolar disorder. Some controversy exists as to whether individuals with bipolar disorder exhibit cognitive styles as negative as those with unipolar depression. A cognitive style named 'anastrophic thinking' has also been described during hypomania [18]. However, it is unclear whether the cognitive changes actually precede or follow mood swings.

Finally, there is a small body of literature addressing the early familial and non-familial environment in the development, expression, and course of bipolar disorder. The evidence is mixed, but there is some suggestion of parenting – characterized by low care and high overprotection, poor attachment relations, and childhood abuse – in the histories of individuals with bipolar disorder. It is also possible that suboptimum parenting and maltreatment may be associated with a worse disease course. But it is also possible that the impact of the illness in one family member might significantly distort family relationships, and cause obvious burden and familial malfunction [19]. Moreover, some relatives might suffer from the condition as well. However, the studies have tended to be small and suffer from major methodological limitations, thus preventing any firm conclusions.

Insights from neuroimaging studies

Recent neuroimaging and postmortem histopathology studies, using techniques such as positron emission tomography, magnetic resonance imaging, single photon emission computed tomography, and magnetic resonance spectroscopy, have identified a range of neurochemical and microstructural differences between brain tissue from bipolar patients and controls (Figure 3.1) [20,21].

There is also evidence for hypothalamic–pituitary–adrenal hyperactivity in depressive phases [22], and some evidence of thyroid dysfunction in bipolar patients with antithyroid antibodies [23]. Deficits have been reported in neural and glial density, measures of glial activity and neuronal integrity, structure, and discrete biochemistry of the frontal cortex, as well as its functional relationships with other areas of the brain. These frontal deficits, together with those in the hippocampus, could account for many of the cognitive deficits observed in the illness and may persist during periods of euthymia [20]. Changes in cerebral

Biochemical, structural, and functional abnormalities in bipolar illness

Biochemical	Structural	Functional	Associativity
Frontal:	↑ Ventricle-to-brain ratio	**Dorsolateral prefrontal cortex**	↓ Cortical/cerebellar reciprocity
↓ Glutamate (layers III–IV)	↑ Hippocampus with greater cognitive impairment	Hypometabolism in bipolar depression	
↓ CaMK-II		Normalizes in mania	
↓ GFAP			
↓ NAA			
↓ Reelin, DLPFC, hippocampus	↓ Glia in subgenual adrenal cortex	Increased cerebellar metabolism (trait)	**Hypersynchrony**
↓ GAD-67	↑ Amygdala	Relative amygdala hypermetabolism at rest	
Anterior cingulate:	↑ Adrenal size	↓ Responsiveness to challenge	
↓ Synaptophysin			
↓ GAP-43			
↓ Complexin II			

Figure 3.1 Biochemical, structural, and functional abnormalities in bipolar illness.
CaMK-II, calcium calmodulin kinase II; DLPFC, dorsolateral prefrontal cortex; GAD, glutamic acid decarboxylase; GAP, growth-associated protein; GFAP, glial fibrillary acidic protein; NAA, N-acetylaspartate. Reproduced with permission from Post et al [20].

volume have been seen in patients with bipolar disorder, but these have not been definitively proven to be a factor in the development of bipolar episodes [24].

Some findings have noted relative baseline increased activity (and perhaps decreased responsivity) of the amygdala and ventral striatum, thalamic imbalance and dysregulation, and relative cerebellar hyperactivity in patients with bipolar disorder. The last is of considerable interest given reports of emotional and affective dysregulation in patients with cerebellar lesions and dysfunction [20,25].

Evidence of diverse and widespread neurological dysfunction in bipolar disorder provides plausible connections between neurobiology and clinical symptoms, particularly bipolar depression (Table 3.1) [26]. However, little is known about how each alteration might be related to the course of illness, either as an underlying cause or as a consequence of episodes and chronicity. Moreover, a comprehensive understanding of the neurobiology of bipolar disorder needs to address the concepts of primary (pathological) versus secondary (adaptive) alterations, as well as differentiating between genetic inheritance versus environmental effects on gene expression (Figure 3.2) [20].

Course of illness

Bipolar disorder is generally an episodic, lifelong illness with a very variable course. The first episode may be manic, hypomanic, mixed, or depressive. Men are more likely than women to be initially manic, but both are more likely to have an index episode of depression [2]. Recent studies suggest that index episode polarity may predict polarity of subsequent episodes [27], and predominant polarity has important clinical and therapeutic implications [28].

In the first decade after diagnosis, the average patient with bipolar disorder will experience around four major mood episodes. The traditional view is that the duration of episodes and interepisode remissions become progressively shorter, before stabilizing after the fourth or fifth episode at around one episode per year [29–31], with an average around one episode per year from disease onset [9]. Only 10–15% of patients are considered 'rapid cyclers', with four or more episodes per year with partial

Features of bipolar depression

Affective

- Sadness
- Apathy
- Anhedonia
- Irritability
- Anxiety

Cognitive

- Poor self-esteem
- Poor concentration
- Indecisiveness
- Suicidal ideas

Physical

- Change in sleep
- Change in appetite
- Decreased activity
- Low energy
- Change in weight

Chemical

- Hypercortisolism
- Decreased somatostatin in cerebrospinal fluid
- Decreased intracellular calcium in blood elements

Brain alterations

- Selective decrease in neurons or glia in prefrontal and anterior cingulated cortex and in amygdala
- Decrease in neuronal NAA in frontal cortex
- Decrease in prefrontal GFAP
- Decreases in reelin and GAD-67
- Frontal and hippocampal hypofunction on PET
- Amygdala and cerebellar hyperactivity on PET
- Loss of normal balance in positive and negative connectivity among brain regions

Table 3.1 Features of bipolar depression. GAD, glutamic acid decarboxylase; GFAP, glial fibrillary acidic protein; NAA, N-acetylaspartate; PET, positron emission tomography. Reproduced with permission from Post [26].

or full remissions in between, or switch to the opposite polarity (manic to depressed, or vice versa) [32]. If untreated, a patient with bipolar disorder is likely to experience more than 10 episodes during their lifetime [2].

Most individuals, over the long term, report fewer manic then depressive episodes. Manic episodes tend to begin abruptly and last for between 2 weeks and 5 months (median: 4 months). Depressions tend to last longer (median: 6 months), though rarely for more than 1 year, and tend to become more common and longer lasting after middle age [2]. It is estimated that a large percentage of patients with

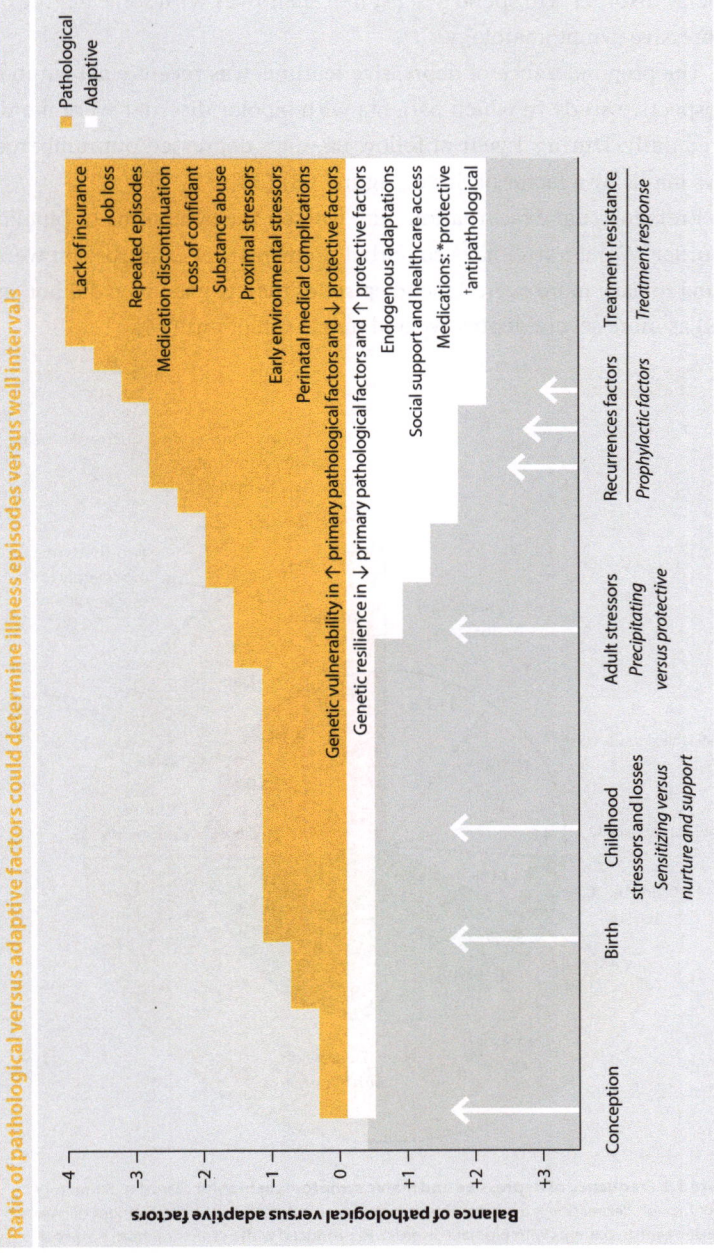

Figure 3.2 Ratio of pathological versus adaptive factors could determine illness episodes versus well intervals. Reproduced with permission from Post et al [20].

bipolar disorder will spend at least half their lives with some degree of depressive symptomatology.

The preponderance of depressive features was recently shown in a prospective study in which patients with bipolar disorder were monitored daily. During 1 year of follow-up, days depressed outnumbered days manic by a factor of three (Figure 3.3) [33].

Premenstrual exacerbation may worsen the symptoms of bipolar disorder. Women who have comorbid premenstrual exacerbation were found to have more overall mood episodes than women who did not, as well as more severe depressive and manic symptoms [34].

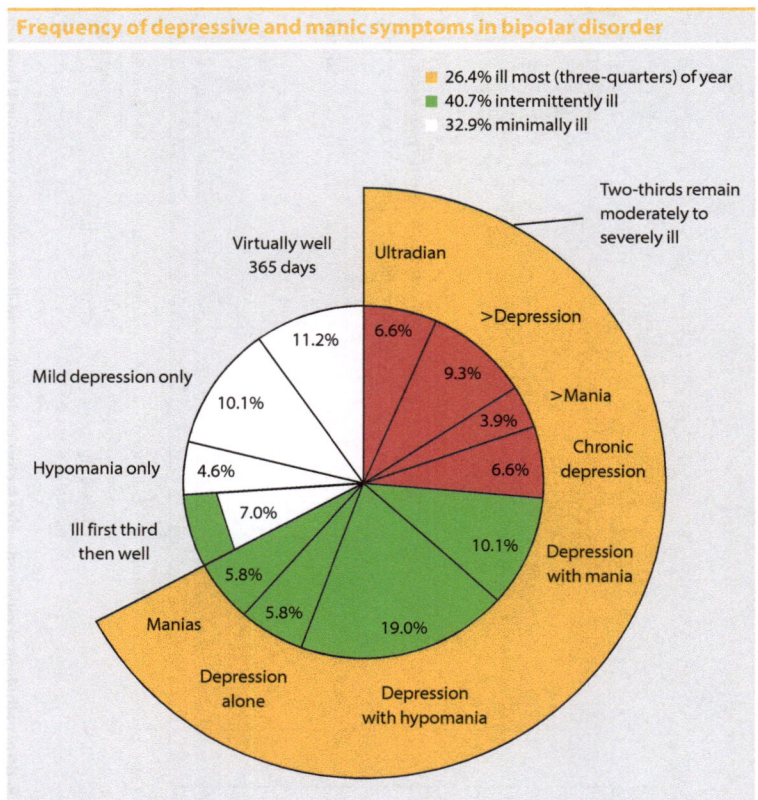

Figure 3.3 Frequency of depressive and manic symptoms in bipolar disorder. Refractory breakthrough depression is a greater problem than mania in the long-term treatment of bipolar disorder, even in patients with bipolar I disorder. Reproduced with permission from Post et al [33].

The US National Institute of Mental Health Collaborative Depression Study offers further insights into the natural history of bipolar disorder. During 15 years of follow-up, the percentage of weeks that bipolar I and II individuals experienced depression was 31% and 52%, respectively. In contrast, they reported hypomania, mania, or mixed episodes in 10% and 1.6% of weeks, respectively. Furthermore, subsyndromal states were three times more common than episodes meeting full syndromal criteria [35,36]. Symptoms of hypomania were seen as a major factor in the progression of patients in the study with unipolar depression to bipolar disorder [37].

In the same study, patients who developed a rapid-cycling pattern suffered substantial depressive morbidity. They were also at very high risk for serious suicide attempts (Table 3.2) [38].

The evidence clearly shows that even patients with frequent severe episodes may also experience long periods with a normal mood state. Although it may be tempting to interpret prolonged periods of wellness as evidence that the diagnosis of bipolar disorder was incorrect, this is seldom the case. The natural history of bipolar disorder often includes periods of remission but, without treatment, bipolar disorder will always relapse. In addition, episodes are often not as discrete, or recoveries as complete, as those described in the diagnostic guidelines. Indeed, much of the disability associated with bipolar disorder stems from the continued

Suicidal behavior in patients with bipolar disorder according to the presence of rapid cycling		
	Any rapid cycling (n=89)	No rapid cycling (n=256)
Before intake	No. (%)	No. (%)
Any attempt	51 (57.3)	85 (33.2)
Any attempt of high intent	31 (34.8)	38 (14.8)
Any attempt of high lethality	36 (40.4)	35 (13.7)
After intake	No. (%)	No. (%)
Completed suicide	3 (3.4)	11 (4.3)
Any attempt	46 (51.7)	70 (27.3)
Any attempt of high intent	27 (30.3)	33 (12.9)
Any attempt of high lethality	30 (33.7)	36 (14.1)

Table 3.2 Suicidal behavior in patients with bipolar disorder according to the presence of rapid cycling. Adapted from Coryell et al [38].

serious impairment experienced during chronic subsyndromal states, as well as subtle cognitive dysfunction [39]. A model has been proposed that integrates the findings from genetic, neurocognitive, and clinical studies (life stressors, progression of illness, medical comorbidity) into the concept of allostatic load. Allostatic load explains the progression of the disease by accumulated neurobiological stress and cognitive impairment, as shown in Figure 3.4 [40].

Signs and symptoms
Mania

The signs and symptoms of mania and hypomania are similar, but in hypomania they are less severe and do not cause significant functional impairment. They include the following:

- increased energy, activity, and restlessness;
- excessively high, overly good, euphoric mood;
- extreme irritability;

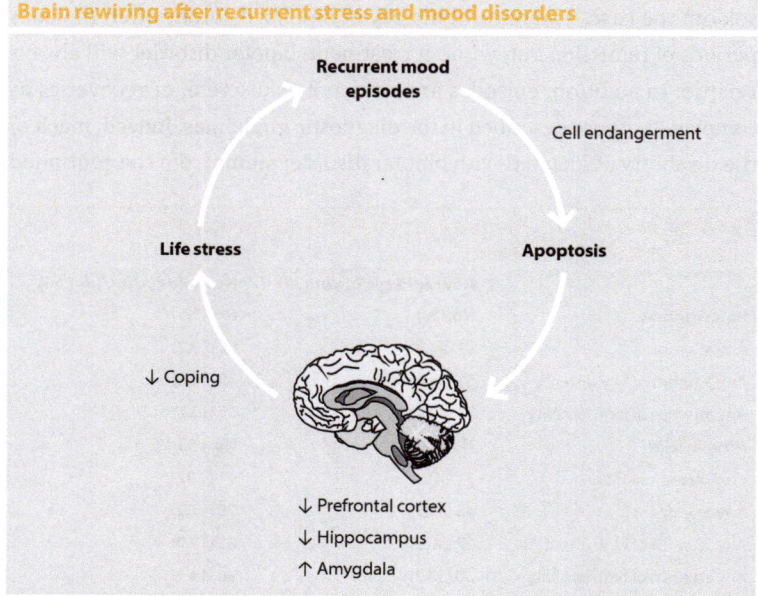

Figure 3.4 Brain rewiring after recurrent stress and mood disorders. Reproduced with permission from Kapczinski et al [40].

- racing thoughts and talking very fast, jumping from one idea to another;
- distractibility, inability to concentrate well;
- little sleep needed;
- unrealistic beliefs in one's abilities and powers;
- poor judgment;
- spending sprees;
- a lasting period of behavior that is different from usual;
- increased sexual drive;
- abuse of drugs, particularly cocaine, alcohol, and sleeping medications;
- provocative, intrusive, or aggressive behavior; and
- denial that anything is wrong.

Depression

The signs and symptoms of depression include the following:
- lasting sad, anxious, or empty mood;
- feelings of hopelessness or pessimism;
- feelings of guilt, worthlessness, or helplessness;
- loss of interest or pleasure in activities once enjoyed, including sex;
- decreased energy, a feeling of fatigue and/or being slowed down;
- restlessness or irritability;
- sleeping too much, or unable to sleep;
- change in appetite and/or unintended weight loss or gain;
- chronic pain or other persistent bodily symptoms not caused by physical illness or injury; and
- thoughts of death or suicide, or suicide attempts.

Psychosis

Severe episodes of mania or depression can include psychotic symptoms, and may lead to people with bipolar disorder being incorrectly diagnosed with schizophrenia [41]. Psychotic symptoms in bipolar disorder often reflect the prevailing mood state (ie, they are mood congruous). For instance, delusions of grandeur may occur during mania, whereas delusions of guilt or worthlessness may appear during depression.

Mood incongruous psychotic experiences can also occur. Psychotic symptoms do not occur in hypomania.

Psychotic symptoms include the following:

- inflated self-esteem;
- hallucinations (hearing, seeing, or otherwise sensing the presence of things that are not actually there and cannot be sensed by others);
- delusions (false, strongly held beliefs not influenced by logical reasoning or explained by a person's usual cultural concepts); and
- inability to communicate due to markedly speeded up, slowed down, or distorted speech (thought disorder, flight of ideas, psychomotor slowing).

Mixed affective states

Symptoms of mania and depression can occur together in a condition called a mixed affective state. Symptoms include agitation, trouble sleeping, significant changes in appetite, psychotic symptoms, and suicidal thinking. The person might have a very sad, hopeless mood while at the same time feeling extremely energized [41]. Agitated depressions are also believed to be mixed states [42].

Early warning signs

Episodes of both mania and depression may be preceded by a prodromal period. These early signs, events, and stressors (sometimes known as the 'relapse signature') can vary from person to person, but typically include a marked increase in the number and magnitude of symptoms compared with remission.

One small study of patients with bipolar disorder found that 85% could identify a depressive prodrome and 75% a manic prodrome. The mean duration of manic prodromes was slightly longer than that of depressive prodromes (28.9 days versus 18.8 days). The majority of patients could identify a time sequence to the retainment of insight during their prodromes and could also identify idiosyncratic symptoms [43].

In a larger series of patients with prospective follow-up, most patients were able to report their prodromal symptoms reliably. In this study, manic prodromes tended to be characterized by behavioral symptoms, while depression prodromes were more diverse and included a mixture of behavioral, cognitive, and somatic symptoms. Common prodromal symptoms in this study are summarized in Table 3.3 [44].

Prognosis

Several recent long-term outcome studies have confirmed the recurrent and often persistent nature of psychopathology in bipolar disorder, with

Common prodromal symptoms of mania and depression reported by patients at T1 and T2		
	Subjects reported at	
	T1 (recruitment) (%)	**T2** (after 18 months) (%)
Mania prodromal symptoms		
Not interested in sleeping or sleeping less	55.3	55.3
More goal-directed behavior (eg, activities with a purpose in mind, such as making more business calls, doing more home improvement projects)	44.7	55.3
Increased sociability	18.4	21.2
Thoughts start to race	15.8	15.8
Irritable	13.2	13.2
Increased optimism	26.3	10.5
Over-excitable and restless	21.1	10.5
Spending too much	13.2	13.2
Increased self-esteem	10.5	15.8
Loss of interest in food	5.3	13.2
Depression prodromal symptoms		
Loss of interest in activity or people	28.9	36.8
Not able to put worries or anxieties aside	18.4	18.4
Interrupted sleep	13.2	26.3
Feeling sad or wanting to cry	15.8	5.3
Low motivation	7.9	10.5
Cannot get out of bed	13.2	13.2
Negative thinking	13.2	7.9
Feeling tired	7.9	26.3
Disinterest in food	7.9	13.2

Table 3.3 Common prodromal symptoms of mania and depression reported by patients at T1 and T2. Adapted from Lam et al [44].

high relapse rates in around three-quarters of patients (Table 3.4) [45]. Interestingly, functional recovery appears to lag behind symptomatic or syndromic recovery, even after a single manic episode [46]. Psychosocial deficits after repeated episodes include lower income and educational or job status versus premorbid levels of impaired social functioning and marital status. In the Chicago Follow-up Study, fewer than half of patients with bipolar disorder had good work functioning during

Summary of findings from recent long-term outcome studies

Study cohort	n	Outcome
NIMH Collaborative Depression Study	113, 146, 86	At 5-year follow-up, bipolar disorder patients showed persistent unemployment, poor job status, and low incomes; at 15-year follow-up, depressive symptoms during the first few follow-up years predicted depressive symptoms at 15-year follow-up, whereas persistent manic symptoms during that time did not predict later manic symptoms; poor functioning before baseline also predicted poor syndromal outcome; and affective symptoms were evident for approximately half the time across follow-up weeks
Chicago Follow-up Study	35	Poorer global, work, and social functioning in bipolar disorder than unipolar disorder; affective relapse was more associated with poorer work functioning among bipolar than unipolar patients; fewer than half of bipolar patients had good work functioning across successive follow-ups over 10 years; and remission at the first two follow-up visits was related to remission at later visits
Pisa, Italy	402	High dropout (about 73%) over 15 years during lithium maintenance was associated with poor outcome; medication adherence was associated with diminished time in hospital during follow-up period
McLean Hospital	75	Over 4 years, poor outcome was associated with prior episode burden, history of comorbid alcohol abuse/dependence, psychosis, male gender, depression symptoms during index manic episode; interepisode affective symptoms at 6-month follow-up predicted poor outcome after index manic episode
UCLA	82	Over 5 years, 73% of patients relapsed into mania or depression during naturalistic pharmacotherapy; of those who relapsed, two-thirds had multiple relapses; poor psychosocial outcome paralleled poor syndromal course; poor psychosocial functioning, especially occupational disruption, predicted a shorter time to relapse. Depressions were most strongly related to social and family dysfunction
McLean– Harvard First Episode Mania Study	166	By 2-year follow-up after an index manic episode, 98% of patients achieved syndromal recovery, 72% had symptomatic recovery, and 43% achieved functional recovery

Table 3.4 Summary of findings from recent long-term outcome studies. NIMH, National Institute of Mental Health; UCLA, University of California, Los Angeles. Reproduced with permission from Goldberg et al [45].

follow-up, and the risk of relapse leading to hospitalization increased with every new episode [47].

Bipolar disorder proves fatal in a high proportion of patients from complications of risk-taking behavior, comorbid medical illnesses, and suicide. A prospective study with over 30 years of follow-up found that standardized mortality rates (observed deaths/expected deaths) were significantly elevated in bipolar patients, with circulatory disorders and suicide being the most frequent causes of death [48].

References

1   Grunze H, Kasper S, Goodwin G, et al. World Federation of Societies of Biological Psychiatry (WFSBP) Guidelines for Biological Treatment of Bipolar Disorders, Part I: Treatment of Bipolar Depression. *World J Biol Psychiatry*. 2002;3:115-124.

2   Hirschfeld RMA, Bowden CL, Perlis RH, et al. American Psychiatric Association. Practice guideline for the treatment of patients with bipolar disorder [Revision]. *Am J Psychiatry*. 2002; 159(4 suppl):1-50.

3   Kendler KS, Pedersen NL, Neale MC, et al. A pilot Swedish twin study of affective illness including hospital- and population-ascertained subsamples: results of model fitting. *Behav Genet*. 1995;25:217-232.

4   Kelsoe JR, Sadovnick AD, Kristbjarnarson H, et al. Possible locus for bipolar disorder near the dopamine transporter on chromosome 5. *Am J Med Genet*. 1996;67:533-540.

5   Waldman ID, Robinson BF, Feigon SA. Linkage disequilibrium between the dopamine transporter gene (DAT1) and bipolar disorder: extending the transmission disequilibrium test (TDT) to examine genetic heterogeneity. *Genet Epidemiol*. 1997;14:699-704.

6   Serretti A, Mandelli L. The genetics of bipolar disorder: genome 'hot regions', genes, new potential candidates and future directions. *Mol Psychiatry*. 2008;13:742-771.

7   Kato T, Kuratomi G, Kato N. Genetics of bipolar disorder. *Drugs Today (Barc)*. 2005;41:335-344.

8   Seifuddin F, Mahon PB, Judy J, et al. Meta-analysis of genetic association studies on bipolar disorder. *Am J Med Genet B Neuropsychiatr Genet*. 2012;159B:508-518.

9   Sanders AR, Duan J, Gejman PV. Complexities in psychiatric genetics. *Int Rev Psychiatry*. 2004;16:284-293.

10   Lichtenstein P, Yip BH, Björk C, et al. Common genetic determinants of schizophrenia and bipolar disorder in Swedish families: a population-based study. *Lancet*. 2009;373:234-239.

11   Pinsonneault JK, Han DD, Burdick KA, et al. Dopamine transporter gene variant affecting expression in human brain is associated with bipolar disorder. *Neuropsychopharmacology*. 2011;36:1644-1655.

12   Sachs G. *Managing Bipolar Affective Disorder*. London, UK: Science Press; 2004.

13   Bertelsen A, Harvald B, Hauge M. A Danish twin study of manic-depressive disorders. *Br J Psychiatry*. 1977;130:330-351.

14   Wehr TA. Sleep-loss as a possible mediator of diverse causes of mania. *Br J Psychiatry*. 1991;159:576-578.

15   Azorin J-M, Angst J, Gamma A, et al. Identifying features of bipolarity in patients with postpartum depression: findings from the international BRIDGE study. *J Affect Disord*. 2010;136:710-715.

16   Alloy LB, Abramson LY, Urosevic S, et al. The psychosocial context of bipolar disorder: environmental, cognitive, and developmental risk factors. *Clin Psychol Rev*. 2005;25:1043-1075.

17 Bauer M, Glenn T, Alda M, et al. Impact of sunlight on the age of onset of bipolar disorder. *Bipolar Disord.* 2012;14:654-663.

18 Colom F, Vieta E. Sudden glory revisited: cognitive contents of hypomania. *Psychother Psychosom.* 2007;76:278-288.

19 Reinares M, Vieta E. The burden on the family of bipolar patients. *Clin Approach Bipolar Disord.* 2004;3:17-23.

20 Post RM, Speer AM, Hough CJ, et al. Neurobiology of bipolar illness: implications for future study and therapeutics. *Ann Clin Psychiatry.* 2003;15:85-94.

21 Phillips ML, Vieta E. Identifying functional neuroimaging biomarkers of bipolar disorder: toward DSM-V. *Schizophr Bull.* 2007;33:893-904.

22 Daban C, Vieta E, Mackin P, et al. Hypothalamic-pituitary-adrenal axis and bipolar disorder. *Psychiatr Clin North Am.* 2005;28:469-480.

23 Kupka RW, Nolen WA, Post RM et al. High rate of autoimmune thyroiditis in bipolar disorder: Lack of association with lithium exposure. *Biol Psychiatry.* 2002;51:305-311.

24 Schneider MR, DelBello MP, McNamara RK, et al. Neuroprogression in bipolar disorder. *Bipolar Disord.* 2012;14:356-374.

25 Schmahmann JD, Sherman JC. The cerebellar cognitive affective syndrome. *Brain.* 1998;121:561-579.

26 Post RM. The impact of bipolar depression. *J Clin Psychiatry.* 2005;66(suppl 5):5-10.

27 Calabrese JR, Vieta E, El-Mallakh R, et al. Mood state at study entry as predictor of the polarity of relapse in bipolar disorder. *Biol Psychiatry.* 2004;56:957-963.

28 Colom F, Vieta E, Daban C, et al. Clinical and therapeutic implications of predominant polarity in bipolar disorder. *J Affect Disord.* 2006;93:13-17.

29 Angst J. The course of affective disorders. In, *Handbook of Biological Psychiatry.* Van Praag HM, Sachar EJ, eds. New York, NY: Marcel Dekker Inc; 1981.

30 Zis AP, Grof P, Webster M, et al. Prediction of relapse in recurrent affective disorder. *Psychopharmacol Bull.* 1980;16:47-49.

31 Roy-Byrne P, Post RM, Uhde TW, et al. The longitudinal course of recurrent affective illness: life chart data from research patients at the NIMH. *Acta Psychiatr Scand Suppl.* 1985;317:1-34.

32 Cruz N, Vieta E, Comes M, et al; the EMBLEM Advisory Board. Rapid-cycling bipolar I disorder: Course and treatment outcome of a large sample across Europe. *J Psychiatr Res.* 2008;42:1068-1075.

33 Post RM, Leverich GS, Altshuler LL, et al. An overview of recent findings of the Stanley Foundations Bipolar Network, pt 1. *Bipolar Disord.* 2003;5:310-319.

34 Dias RS, Lafer B, Russo C, et al. Longitudinal follow-up of bipolar disorder in women with premenstrual exacerbation: findings from STEP-BD. *Am J Psychiatry.* 2011;168:386-394.

35 Judd LL, Akiskal HS, Schettler PJ, et al. A prospective investigation of the natural history of the long-term weekly symptomatic status of bipolar II disorder. *Arch Gen Psychiatry.* 2003;60:261-269.

36 Judd LL, Akiskal HS, Schettler PJ et al. The long-term natural history of the weekly symptomatic status of bipolar I disorder. *Arch Gen Psychiatry.* 2002;59:530-537.

37 Fiedorowicz JG, Endicott J, Leon AC, et al. Subthreshold hypomanic symptoms in progression from unipolar major depression to bipolar disorder. *Am J Psychiatry.* 2011;168:40-48.

38 Coryell W, Solomon D, Turvey C, et al. The long-term course of rapid-cycling bipolar disorder. *Arch Gen Psychiatry.* 2003;60:914-920.

39 Martinez-Aran A, Vieta E, Colom F, et al. Cognitive impairment in euthymic bipolar patients: implications for clinical and functional outcome. *Bipolar Disord.* 2004;6:224-232.

40 Kapczinski F, Vieta E, Andreazza AC, et al. Allostatic load in bipolar disorder: implications for pathophysiology and treatment. *Neurosci Biobehav Rev.* 2008;32:675-692.

41 Spearing M. *Bipolar Disorder.* 2nd ed. Bethesda, MD: National Institute of Mental Health; 2001.

42 Benazzi F, Koukopoulos A, Akiskal HS. Toward a validation of a new definition of agitated depression as a bipolar mixed state (mixed depression). *Eur Psychiatry.* 2004;19:85-90.

43 Smith JA, Tarrier N. Prodromal symptoms in manic depressive psychosis. *Soc Psychiatry Psychiatr Epidemiol.* 1992;27:245-248.

44 Lam D, Wong G, Sham P. Prodromes, coping strategies and course of illness in bipolar affective disorder – a naturalistic study. *Psychol Med.* 2001;31:1397-1402.

45 Goldberg JF, Garno JL, Harrow M. Long-term remission and recovery in bipolar disorder: a review. *Curr Psychiatry Rep.* 2005;7:456-461.

46 Tohen M, Zarate CA Jr, Hennen J, et al. The McLean–Harvard First Episode Mania Study: prediction of recovery and first recurrence. *Am J Psychiatry.* 2003;160:2099-2107.

47 Goldberg JF, Harrow M. Consistency of remission and outcome in bipolar and unipolar mood disorders: a 10-year prospective follow-up. *J Affect Disord.* 2004;81:123-131.

48 Angst F, Stassen HH, Clayton PJ, et al. Mortality of patients with mood disorders: follow-up over 34–38 years. *J Affect Disord.* 2002;68:167-0181.

Chapter 4

Assessment and diagnosis

Criteria for diagnosis

The diagnosis of bipolar disorder relies on clinical assessment, augmented by the use of screening tools and diagnostic scales. Two diagnostic schemes are used: the ICD-10 [1,2] and the DSM-IV-TR [3].

The Structured Clinical Interview for DSM (SCID) is the standard research tool to identify bipolar disorder according to the DSM-IV-TR criteria [4], whereas the Present State Examination can be used for ICD-10 diagnostic coding [5]. Screening tools are discussed in more detail below.

DSM-IV-TR

According to the DSM-IV-TR, patients with bipolar I disorder have had at least one episode of mania (Table 4.1) [6]. Some patients have had previous depressive episodes (Table 4.2), and most patients will have subsequent episodes that are either manic or depressive. Hypomanic and mixed episodes (Tables 4.3 and 4.4) may also occur, as can significant subthreshold mood lability between episodes [6]. By contrast, patients meeting criteria for bipolar II disorder have a history of major depressive episodes (MDEs) and hypomanic episodes only. Clinical differences between bipolar I and bipolar II disorders are summarized in Table 4.5 [6,7].

A subanalysis of the BRIDGE study reviewed the DSM-IV-TR criteria for hypomania in the context of patients treated for MDEs and assessed for bipolar disorder. They found that criterion B would exclude a hypomania diagnosis in 80% of their patients who presented with irritable mood

E. Vieta, *Managing Bipolar Disorder in Clinical Practice*,
DOI: 10.1007/978-1-908517-94-4_4, © Springer Healthcare 2013

DSM-IV-TR diagnostic criteria for a manic episode

A. A distinct period of abnormally and persistently elevated, expansive, or irritable mood, lasting at least 1 week (or any duration if hospitalization is necessary)

B. During the period of mood disturbance, three (or more) of the following symptoms have persisted (four if the mood is only irritable) and have been present to a significant degree:
- inflated self-esteem or grandiosity;
- decreased need for sleep (eg, feels rested after only 3 hours of sleep);
- more talkative than usual or pressure to keep talking;
- flight of ideas or subjective experience that thoughts are racing;
- distractibility (ie, attention too easily drawn to unimportant or irrelevant external stimuli);
- increase in goal-directed activity (either socially, at work or school, or sexually) or psychomotor agitation; and
- excessive involvement in pleasurable activities that have a high potential for painful consequences (eg, engaging in unrestrained buying sprees, sexual indiscretions, or foolish business investments)

C. The symptoms do not meet the criteria for a mixed episode

D. The mood disturbance:
- is sufficiently severe to cause marked impairment in occupational functioning, usual social activities, or relationships with others;
- necessitates hospitalization to prevent harm to self or others; and
- has psychotic features

E. The symptoms are not due to the direct physiological effects of a substance (eg, a drug of abuse, a medication, or other treatment) or a general medical condition (eg, hyperthyroidism)

Table 4.1 DSM-IV-TR diagnostic criteria for a manic episode. Manic-like episodes that are clearly caused by somatic antidepressant treatment (eg, medication, electroconvulsive therapy, light therapy) should not count toward a diagnosis of bipolar I disorder. Reproduced with permission from the American Psychiatric Association [6].

and 50% of patients who presented with euphoria or increased activity. More patients had hypomania symptoms for less than 3 days than for 4 or more days; therefore, they would not fulfill criterion A. The authors concluded that a broader definition of hypomania/bipolar II disorder would allow for earlier diagnosis and treatment [8,9].

Some patients may exhibit significant evidence of mood lability and affective symptoms but fail to meet duration criteria for bipolar II disorder, thereby leading to a diagnosis of bipolar disorder, not otherwise specified. Diagnostic features include very rapid alternation between manic and depressive symptoms, recurrent hypomania without intercurrent depressive symptoms, manic or mixed episodes superimposed on delusional or psychotic disorder, and bipolar disorder of uncertain etiology (ie, unable to determine if primary, substance induced, or related to a medical condition).

DSM-IV-TR diagnostic criteria for a major depressive episode

A. Five (or more) of the following symptoms have been present nearly every day during the same 2-week period and represent a change from previous functioning; at least one of the symptoms is either depressed mood or loss of interest or pleasure:

- depressed mood* most of the day as indicated by either subjective report (eg, feels sad or empty) or observation made by others (eg, appears tearful);
- markedly diminished interest or pleasure in all, or almost all, activities most of the day (as indicated by either subjective account or observation made by others);
- significant weight loss when not dieting†,weight gain (eg, a change of >5% body weight in 1 month), or a decrease or increase in appetite;
- insomnia or hypersomnia;
- psychomotor agitation or retardation (observable by others, not merely subjective feelings of restlessness or being slowed down);
- fatigue or loss of energy;
- feelings of worthlessness or excessive or inappropriate guilt (which may be delusional)‡
- diminished ability to think or concentrate or indecisiveness (either by subjective account or as observed by others); and
- recurrent thoughts of death (not just fear of dying), recurrent suicidal ideation without a specific plan, or previous suicide attempt or a specific plan for committing suicide

B. The symptoms do not meet the criteria for a mixed episode

C. The symptoms cause clinically significant distress or impairment in social, occupational, or other important areas of functioning

D. The symptoms are not due to the direct physiological effects of a substance (eg, a drug of abuse, a medication) or a general medical condition (eg, hypothyroidism)

E. The symptoms are not better accounted for by bereavement (ie, after the loss of a loved one) and have persisted for longer than 2 months or are characterized by marked functional impairment, morbid preoccupation with worthlessness, suicidal ideation, psychotic symptoms, or psychomotor retardation

Table 4.2 DSM-IV-TR diagnostic criteria for a major depressive episode. Mood-incongruent delusions, hallucinations, and symptoms that are clearly due to a general medical condition should not count toward a diagnosis of major depressive disorder. *In children and adolescents, mood can also be irritable. †In children, can also include failure to make expected weight gains. ‡Symptoms extend beyond mere self-reproach or guilt about being sick. Reproduced with permission from the American Psychiatric Association [6].

Finally, cyclothymic disorder may be diagnosed in patients who have never experienced a manic, mixed, or major depressive episode but who experience numerous periods of depressive symptoms and numerous periods of hypomanic symptoms for at least 2 years (1 year in children), with no asymptomatic period lasting longer than 2 months.

The subtypes of bipolar disorder, as well as other affective illnesses, are summarized and compared in Table 4.6 [6].

In addition to providing definitions of bipolar disorder, DSM-IV-TR also includes specifiers describing the course of recurrent episodes, such as seasonal pattern, longitudinal course (with or without full interepisode recovery), and rapid cycling.

DSM-IV-TR diagnostic criteria for a hypomanic episode

A. A distinct period of persistently elevated, expansive, or irritable mood, lasting at least 4 days, that is clearly different from the usual non-depressed mood

B. During the period of mood disturbance, three (or more) of the following symptoms have persisted (four if the mood is only irritable) and have been present to a significant degree:
  - inflated self-esteem or grandiosity
  - decreased need for sleep (eg, feels rested after only 3 hours of sleep)
  - more talkative than usual or pressure to keep talking
  - flight of ideas or subjective experience that thoughts are racing
  - distractibility (ie, attention too easily drawn to unimportant or irrelevant external stimuli)
  - increase in goal-directed activity (either socially, at work or school, or sexually) or psychomotor agitation
  - excessive involvement in pleasurable activities that have a high potential for painful consequences (eg, engaging in unrestrained buying sprees, sexual indiscretions, or foolish business investments)

C. The episode is associated with an unequivocal change in functioning that is uncharacteristic of the person when not symptomatic

D. The disturbance in mood and the change in functioning are observable by others

E. The episode:
  - is not severe enough to cause marked impairment in social or occupational functioning
  - does not necessitate hospitalization
  - does not have psychotic features

F. The symptoms are not due to the direct physiological effects of a substance (eg, a drug of abuse, a medication, or other treatment) or a general medical condition (eg, hyperthyroidism)

Table 4.3 DSM-IV-TR diagnostic criteria for a hypomanic episode. Hypomanic-like episodes that are clearly caused by somatic antidepressant treatment (eg, medication, electroconvulsive therapy, light therapy) should not count toward a diagnosis of bipolar II disorder. Reproduced with permission from the American Psychiatric Association [6].

Diagnostic criteria for a mixed episode

A. The criteria are met both for a manic episode and for a major depressive episode (except for duration) nearly every day during at least a 1-week period

B. The mood disturbance:
  - is sufficiently severe to cause marked impairment in occupational functioning, usual social activities, or relationships with others
  - necessitates hospitalization to prevent harm to self or others
  - has psychotic features

C. The symptoms are not due to the direct physiological effects of a substance (eg, a drug of abuse, a medication, or other treatment) or a general medical condition (eg, hyperthyroidism)

Table 4.4 Diagnostic criteria for a mixed episode. Mixed-like episodes that are clearly caused by somatic antidepressant treatment (eg, medication, electroconvulsive therapy, light therapy) should not count toward a diagnosis of bipolar I disorder. Reproduced with permission from the American Psychiatric Association [6].

Clinical differences between bipolar I and bipolar II disorder

Clinical feature	Bipolar I	Bipolar II
Symptom profile	More severe symptoms	Less severe acute symptoms
	Hospitalization due to mania	Depressive symptoms likely to predominate Hospitalization due to depression
Clinical course	More likely to experience hypomania	More chronic course with more episodes of longer duration
Comorbidity	More comorbidities than the general population	More comobordities than the general population
Switching frequency	May be less frequent than bipolar II	May be more frequent than bipolar I

Table 4.5 Clinical differences between bipolar I and bipolar II disorder. Adapted from Suppes et al [7].

Summary of manic and depressive symptom criteria in DSM-IV-TR mood disorders

Disorder	Manic symptom criteria	Depressive criteria
Major depressive disorder	No history of mania or hypomania	History of major depressive episodes (single or recurrent)
Dysthymic disorder	No history of mania or hypomania	Depressed mood, more days than not, for at least 2 years (but not meeting criteria for a major depressive episode)
Bipolar I disorder	History of manic or mixed episodes	Major depressive episodes are typical but are not required for diagnosis
Bipolar II disorder	One or more episodes of hypomania; no manic or mixed episodes	History of major depressive episodes
Cyclothymic disorder	For at least 2 years, the presence of numerous periods with hypomanic symptoms	Numerous periods with depressive symptoms that do not meet criteria for a major depressive episode
Bipolar disorder not otherwise specified	Manic symptoms present, but criteria not met for bipolar I, bipolar II, or cyclothymic disorder	Not required for diagnosis

Table 4.6 Summary of manic and depressive symptom criteria in DSM-IV-TR mood disorders. Reproduced with permission from the American Psychiatric Association [6].

ICD-10

The ICD-10 diagnostic criteria are mostly equivalent to those of DSM-IV-TR, although there is no distinction between bipolar I and bipolar II disorders. ICD-10 defines bipolar affective disorder as multiple episodes of mania/hypomania, or both depression and mania/hypomania, as well as specifying the nature of the current episode. The ICD-10 scheme divides depressive episodes according to their severity (mild, moderate, severe). It also classifies both manic and severe depressive episodes as with or without psychotic symptoms. The key features of the ICD-10 scheme are highlighted below [10].

Hypomania

Persistent mild elevation or irritability of mood for at least 4 days. At least three of the following are present:

- increased energy and activity;
- increased sociability;
- talkativeness;
- over-familiarity;
- mild overspending or other types of recklessness and irresponsible behavior;
- increased sexual energy;
- decreased need for sleep; and
- difficulty in concentration or distractibility.

Symptoms may lead to moderate, but not severe, disruption of work or result in social rejection. The disturbances of mood and behavior are not accompanied by hallucinations or delusions.

Mania without psychotic symptoms

For at least 1 week (or less if hospitalized): mood elevation, expansive, or irritable out of keeping with the patient's circumstances.

At least three of the following are present:

- increased activity or physical restlessness;
- pressure of speech;
- flight of ideas or racing thoughts;
- loss of normal social inhibitions;
- decreased need for sleep;
- distractibility or constant changes in plans;
- inflated self-esteem with grandiose ideas and overconfidence;
- behavior that is foolhardy and reckless; and
- marked sexual energy or indiscretion.

Mania with psychotic symptoms

As mania without psychotic symptoms, but in addition: delusions (usually grandiose) or hallucinations (usually of voices speaking directly to the patient), excessive motor activity, and flight of ideas that are so extreme that the person is incomprehensible or inaccessible to ordinary communication.

Mixed episode

The patient has had at least one authenticated hypomanic, manic, depressive, or mixed affective episode in the past, and currently exhibits either a mixture or a rapid alteration of manic and depressive symptoms.

Depressive episode

For at least 2 weeks: lowering of mood, reduction of energy, and decrease in activity. Capacity for enjoyment, interest, and concentration is reduced, and marked tiredness even after minimum effort is common. Sleep is usually disturbed and appetite diminished. Self-esteem and self-confidence are almost always reduced and, even in the mild form, ideas of guilt or worthlessness are often present. Low mood varies little from day to day, is unresponsive to circumstances, and may be accompanied by somatic symptoms such as loss of interest in pleasure, waking in the morning before the usual time, depression worst in the morning, marked psychomotor retardation, agitation, loss of appetite, weight loss, and loss of libido.

Depressive episodes may be specified as mild (at least four symptoms), moderate (at least six symptoms and difficulty performing ordinary activities), or severe (at least eight symptoms, symptoms are marked and distressing).

Severe depressive episodes are specified as with or without psychotic symptoms, with psychotic symptoms defined as the presence of delusions, hallucinations, or depressive stupor. Auditory or olfactory hallucinations are usually of defamatory or accusatory voices or of rotting filth or decomposing flesh. Severe psychomotor retardation may progress to stupor. If required, delusions or hallucinations may be specified as mood congruent or mood incongruent.

Diagnostic challenges

Misdiagnosis and underdiagnosis

Diagnosing bipolar disorder can be a challenge, and delays of up to 20 years between the onset of symptoms and initiation of treatment have been reported [6]. Delays in diagnosis may be associated with instability of presentation. For instance, in a cohort of patients experiencing a first psychotic episode, only 75% of patients retained their initial diagnosis of bipolar disorder after 6 months [10]. Bipolar disorder, however, happened to be the most stable diagnosis in a large cohort of 500 patients with first-episode psychosis in the McLean-Harvard First Episode Project [11].

A survey of 600 patients with bipolar disorder found that two-thirds were initially misdiagnosed; the incorrect diagnoses included major depressive disorder, anxiety disorder, schizophrenia, and personality disorder. In this study, one-third of respondents experienced a delay of more than 10 years between first consultation and accurate diagnosis. Those who were misdiagnosed consulted an average of four physicians and received an average of 3.5 different incorrect diagnoses [12].

Factors that can confound the diagnostic process include overlapping symptomatology, particularly with major depressive disorder (unipolar depression), comorbidities (especially anxiety and substance use disorders), and the late occurrence of manic or hypomanic symptoms in patients with recurrent depressive illness. It is estimated that 35–45% of patients with bipolar I disorder are misdiagnosed with unipolar depression. One of the reasons for this is that patients with bipolar disorder seek treatment in the depressive state two to three times more often than in the manic state [6]. Another factor is that many patients with hypomania regard their symptoms as normal or desirable, and therefore underreport them [13]. Applying the DSM-IV-TR and bipolarity criteria to patients in treatment for major depressive disorder may help identify early on those who may be at risk of developing bipolar disorder [14].

A major consequence of the failure to accurately identify and diagnose patients with bipolar disorder is to worsen their long-term prognosis. Delayed diagnosis allows complications and comorbidities, including substance misuse, to progress [7,15]. Furthermore, pharmacological and psychosocial treatments for bipolar disorder may be less effective in patients who have experienced several untreated or inappropriately treated episodes [16,17].

Conversely, it is important to exclude the possibility of a bipolar diagnosis in all patients who present initially with depressive symptoms in order to avoid inappropriate treatment. The use of antidepressant monotherapy in patients with bipolar disorder may induce a manic episode in 30–40% of individuals [18]. There may also be a risk of inducing rapid cycling, which is associated with increased treatment resistance and worse outcomes [19]. One study assessed the occurrence of mixed episodes during follow-up in patients with bipolar I disorder treated with antidepressants. Nearly 42% experienced at least one mixed episode, and that group had higher switch rates and relapse rates compared with those who had not had a mixed episode. They also had a longer average duration of illness and greater number of total episodes [20].

To avoid these complications, current clinical practice guidelines recommend the prescription of an antidepressant, if appropriate, to be taken in combination of a mood stabiliser in bipolar disorder patients [6,21]. Delaying the introduction of a mood stabiliser may increase the risk of lithium resistance [22], suicide [23,24], and substance abuse [25]. However, even the combination of an antidepressant with another agent has been associated with depressive polarity of the most recent episode during the maintenance phase [26].

The US Food and Drug Administration (FDA) was sufficiently concerned about the inappropriate use of antidepressant monotherapy in bipolar disorder patients to include a specific warning in a Public Health Advisory in 2004 [27]. It states:

> " Because antidepressants are believed to have the potential for inducing manic episodes in patients with bipolar disorder, there is a concern about using antidepressants alone in this population. Therefore, patients should be adequately screened to determine if they are at risk for bipolar disorder before initiating antidepressant treatment so that they can be appropriately monitored during treatment. "

Antidepressant use is of particular concern in adolescent and young adult patients. In 2007, the FDA issued a recommendation that the black box warning for all antidepressants include warnings on the increased risk of suicidality in patients aged 18 to 24 years during the first two months of treatment [28].

Further research is urgently needed to clarify the potential role and risks of antidepressant use in bipolar disorder [29,30]. Unfortunately, antidepressants are still the most frequently prescribed drugs in patients with bipolar disorder [31,32]. Physicians need to be aware of the benefits and risks of treating bipolar disorder with antidepressants as well as potential alternative therapies for depression [32].

Although underdiagnosis of bipolar disorder is very common world-wide, there have been recently voices claiming that the US may have gone too far trying to correct that trend, and that bipolar disorder might be overdiagnosed [33], particularly in children and adolescents [34]. It is also important to distinguish between the manic phase of bipolar disorder and attention deficit hyperactivity disorder (ADHD), as they present with similar symptoms. However, ADHD is characterized by over-talkativeness, distractibility, and restlessness [35].

Differential diagnosis

Clinical features that may distinguish between unipolar and bipolar depression are summarized in Table 4.7, while clinical features suggestive

Clinical features that may distinguish between major depressive disorder (unipolar depression) and bipolar depression	
Unipolar depression	**Bipolar depression**
Typically emerges after the age of 25 years	Typically emerges before the age of 25 years
	Episodes may be abrupt in onset (hours or days)
May be preceded by an extended period of gradually worsening symptoms	Often periodic or seasonal
	Treatment-emergent mania/hypomania during antidepressant monotherapy may be suggestive of bipolarity
No history of mania or hypomania	Highly heritable; bipolar disorder often runs in families, and a thorough family history is a vital diagnostic step
	A history of mania, hypomania, or increased energy and decreased need for sleep

Table 4.7 Clinical features that may distinguish between major depressive disorder (unipolar depression) and bipolar depression. Reproduced with permission from Suppes et al [7].

of bipolarity in patients presenting with depressive symptoms are given in Table 4.8 [7].

Many other conditions can produce symptoms similar to those seen in bipolar disorder, including general medical conditions, alcohol and substance abuse, medications, and psychiatric disorders including schizophrenia. Conditions to consider in the differential diagnosis of depressive and manic syndromes, as well as their distinguishing features, are summarized in Table 4.9 [36].

Screening tools

A number of strategies can be used to screen for bipolar disorder in clinical practice. These include eliciting a full history of symptoms from the patient, obtaining collateral information from family and friends, and the prospective use of a mood diary. Factors to consider when considering a diagnosis of bipolar disorder are summarized in Table 4.10 [36].

For the busy physician with limited time, screening questionnaires and rating scales can be very useful. There is no 'gold standard' screening tool, but several scales are relevant in diagnosing bipolar disorder [37] and are discussed in brief below.

Clinical features that may suggest bipolarity in patients presenting with depressive symptoms	
Clinical feature	Explanation
A history of antidepressant failures	Failure to respond to three or more adequate trials of unimodal antidepressants
Antidepressant-induced activation	Activation of symptoms such as restlessness, irritability, and insomnia, particularly in patients initially diagnosed with panic disorder or generalized anxiety disorder
Behavioral disruptions	Patients exhibiting disruptive behavioral patterns should be assessed for both bipolar disorder and axis II personality disorder
History of manic/hypomanic symptoms	Patients presenting with depressive symptoms often fail to recall or recognize periods of mania/hypomania, and input from significant others/caregivers may prove useful. Education directed at helping patients recognize past of current hypomania is important

Table 4.8 Clinical features that may suggest bipolarity in patients presenting with depressive symptoms. Adapted from Suppes et al [7].

Differential diagnosis of bipolar disorder

Diagnosis	Distinguishing features
Major depressive or dysthymic disorder	Manic or hypomanic episodes probed for and not present
Mood disorder due to a general medical condition	Episodes are judged to be a consequence of a medical condition such as multiple sclerosis, stroke or hyperthyroidism. Onset or exacerbation of mood coincides with that of medical condition
Substance-induced mood disorder	Episodes are judged to be a consequence of a substance such as an illicit drug, a medication (stimulants, steroids, l-dopa, antidepressants), or toxin exposure. Episodes may be related to intoxication or withdrawal
Cyclothymic disorder	Hypomanic symptoms do not meet the criteria for a manic episode, and depressive symptoms do not meet the criteria for a major depressive episode
Psychotic disorders (schizoaffective disorder, schizophrenia, delusional disorder)	Periods of psychotic symptoms in the absence of prominent mood symptoms. Consider onset, accompanying symptoms, previous course, and family history
Borderline personality disorder	Instability of interpersonal relationships, self-image, and mood, with marked impulsivity, and a central theme of intense abandonment fears. Early onset and a long-standing course. True euphoria and prolonged well-functioning intervals are extremely rare
Narcissistic personality disorder	Grandiosity, need for admiration, and lack of empathy of early onset. Grandiosity not associated with mood changes or functional impairments
Antisocial personality disorder	Early onset of disregard for, and violation of, the rights of others, which does not occur only in the context of a manic episode

Table 4.9 Differential diagnosis of bipolar disorder. Reproduced with permission from Yatham et al [36].

Mood Disorder Questionnaire

The Mood Disorder Questionnaire (MDQ) screens for a lifetime history of manic or hypomanic symptoms. It does not distinguish between the different types of bipolar disorder, but is probably most sensitive at detecting bipolar I disorder. It is especially useful in primary care; patients who screen positive on the MDQ should then receive a complete clinical assessment for bipolar spectrum disorder. The MDQ can be completed by the patient or clinical staff in less than 5 minutes [38]. It is important to note that the MDQ should only be used as a screening tool and not as

Interviewing for the potential of bipolar disorder

Who to screen?

- Screen patients who present with depressive symptoms for a history of hypomanic or manic symptoms
- Consider an underlying mood disorder in patients presenting with unexplained vague/non-specific somatic symptoms or reverse vegetative symptoms (eg, hypersomnia and hyperphagia)

How to screen?

- Listen to the patient's unprompted presenting complaints
- Ask open-ended and non-leading general questions about the common symptoms of depression and mania
- Ask questions about specific symptoms of depression and mania, including how long the symptoms have been present during the current episode, how long they lasted during prior episodes (if applicable), and whether they have caused problems in social relationships or work
- Always ask about suicidal ideation
- Ask about psychotic symptoms
- Consider asking the patient to complete the Mood Disorder Questionnaire
- Ask about a family history of bipolar disorder
- Interview family or friends regarding prior episodes of mania or hypomania
- If unclear, ask patients to do prospective mood ratings and assess when patients are rating symptoms in manic or hypomanic range

Consider alternative diagnoses

- General medical conditions that may produce similar symptoms
- Alcohol and other substance abuse
- Medications that may produce similar symptoms

Table 4.10 Interviewing for the potential of bipolar disorder. Reproduced with permission from Yatham et al [36].

a diagnostic proxy or a case-finding measure, even though it has been used that way in several clinical trials. This is due to its relatively low sensitivity and small positive predictive value [39].

Bipolar Spectrum Diagnostic Scale

The Bipolar Spectrum Diagnostic Scale (BSDS) is a screening instrument for bipolar disorder and was designed to capture the more subtle features of bipolar II disorder. It is a narrative account of 19 features that may occur in people with bipolar disorder. The narrative is read by the patient who rates it for overall applicability to their particular situation, before rating each feature individually [40]. Patients identified with probable or possible bipolar disorder should undergo a comprehensive diagnostic evaluation, eg, using a recognized diagnostic system such as the SCID and obtaining a collateral history from a close friend or family member.

Beck Depression Inventory

The Beck Depression Inventory (BDI) was introduced in 1961 and has become one of the most widely used depression rating scales [41]. It is a 21-item self-administered scale that takes about 10 minutes to complete. The inventory covers a range of somatic, cognitive, affective, and behavioral symptoms associated with depression. It can be used as a screening tool and has been shown to discriminate effectively between depressed and non-depressed individuals. It is useful for monitoring response to treatment, but is less effective at gauging the severity of a depressive episode.

Montgomery and Asberg Depression Rating Scale

The Montgomery and Asberg Depression Rating Scale (MADRS) is a 10-item depression rating scale [42]. It has been used widely in clinical trials of antidepressant medication for quantitative evaluation and assessment of changes in symptoms. There is a relative lack of emphasis on somatic symptoms compared with other depression rating scales, making it particularly useful for the assessment of depression in people with physical illnesses. It is administered by a trained interviewer, has good inter-rater reliability, and takes approximately 15–20 minutes. Due to higher sensitivity than the Hamilton Depression Rating Scale (HAM-D or HDRS) in some studies [43], it is becoming the preferred outcome measure for depressive symptoms in clinical trials on patients with bipolar disorder.

Hamilton Depression Rating Scale

The HAM-D has been described as the gold standard of observer-completed depression rating scales [44,45]. It is a well-validated and highly reliable scale that has been extensively used in clinical research, including clinical trials of antidepressant drugs. Similar to the MADRS scale, the HAM-D is a semi-structured interview; however, the latter has more emphasis on the patient report than the direct observations of the interviewer. Additional information from nursing staff, family, or friends can also be taken into account. It takes approximately 30 minutes to complete and should be administered by a trained interviewer.

Clinician-Administered Rating Scale for Mania

The Clinician-Administered Rating Scale for Mania (CARS-M) is a 15-item scale that screens for mania in the previous 7 days. It is used to assess the severity of a manic episode, including psychotic symptoms, to assist diagnosis by identifying the presence of manic symptoms (individual items correspond to DSM-IV-TR diagnostic criteria for mania), and to assess response to antimania treatment in clinical trials [46].

Young Mania Rating Scale

The Young Mania Rating Scale (YMRS) is a reliable 11-item clinician-administered rating scale used to assess the severity of mania for either clinical or research purposes [47]. It is scored by the interviewer based on the subjective reports of the patient, coupled with the interviewer's own observations of the patient's behavior during the interview. The major drawbacks of the scale are that it assesses only manic symptoms (there are no items assessing depression), it may be difficult to administer in patients who are highly thought disordered, and it may not be as sensitive for mild forms of mania, such as hypomania. However, it has become the standard measure for clinical trials in mania.

Hypomania Checklist

The Hypomania Checklist (HCL-32) is a 32-item checklist that helps identify patients with bipolar II disorder who might otherwise be classified as suffering from an MDE (major depressive episode) [48]. It may also be useful in the identification of patients with minor bipolar disorders (eg, hypomanic symptoms in the presence of dysthymia, minor depression, or recurrent brief depression). Because the HCL is administered by the patient, it has distinct advantages over lengthy structured interviews such as the SCID, and thus represents a useful tool for the busy clinician. It may also be slightly more sensitive than the MDQ [49].

Special considerations
Children and adolescents

The assessment of bipolar disorder in certain patient groups, such as children and adolescents, poses specific diagnostic challenges. It is estimated that 53–66% of patients experience their first episode during childhood or adolescence, with a peak age of onset between 15 and 19 years [50]. The prevalence of bipolar disorder in a community sample of 14 to 18 year olds was 1%, with a further 5.7% meeting criteria for bipolar disorder, not otherwise specified [51]. Around 20% of children diagnosed with major depressive disorder subsequently experience manic episodes [52]. Of note, the earlier the onset of bipolar disorder the greater the likelihood of suicide attempts [53].

Diagnosing childhood bipolar disorder is complicated by the high rates of psychiatric comorbidity, including attention deficit hyperactivity disorder (ADHD), dysthymia, anxiety, and conduct disorders. An estimated 88% of bipolar children have another psychiatric disorder and 76% a comorbid anxiety disorder [54]. In one study, 91% of children with current or past mania also met criteria for ADHD, which has been associated with a poorer response to therapy [55]. The following are factors to consider in the differential diagnosis of early onset bipolar disorder and ADHD [36]:

- True euphoria, decreased need for sleep and hypersexuality are common in bipolar disorder, but uncommon in ADHD.
- The onset of symptoms (including inattention) usually occurs in individuals over 7 years of age in bipolar disorder, but begins earlier in ADHD.
- Family history of bipolar disorder is more common with bipolar disorder, whereas disruptive disorders (ie, conduct disorder) is more frequently seen in individuals with ADHD.
- Periods of normal functioning may be seen in those with bipolar disorder, but is infrequent in individuals with ADHD.

Although the DSM-IV-TR or ICD-10 criteria are used to diagnose bipolar disorder in childhood and adolescence, children with mania often present with atypical symptoms [36], including:

- erratic, not persistent, changes in mood, their level of psychomotor agitation, and mental excitement;
- irritability, belligerence, and mixed state – these are more commonly seen than euphoria;
- reckless behavior, such as school failure, fighting, dangerous play, or inappropriate sexual activity;

- psychotic symptoms, mood incongruent hallucinations, paranoia, marked thought disorder; and
- severe deterioration in behavior.

Around half of children with mood lability and sleep disturbance early in life meet all DSM-IV-TR criteria except the episode duration requirements [56]. These atypical and complicated presentations have led to the underdiagnosis of bipolar disorder in teenagers and misdiagnosis as schizophrenia. A diagnosis of bipolar disorder should be considered in any individual with a marked deterioraton in functioning associated with either mood or psychotic symptoms. It is very important to correctly diagnose bipolar disorder and diagnose it early. An inverse relationship has been shown between age of onset and delay of first treatment, and a earlier treatment delay is a prognostic factor of poorer outcome later in life, along with early disease onset [15].

Useful diagnostic tools for pediatric bipolar disorder include the Child Behavior Checklist [57], the Young Mania Rating Scale – Parent Version [58], the Children's Global Assessment Scale [59], and the Washington University in St Louis Kiddie Schedule for Affective Disorders and Schizophrenia [60,61]. The diagnosis of bipolar disorder in children and adolescents has increased 40-fold in a decade and there is an ongoing debate on the extent to which this increment reflects a true augmentation of the incidence of the disorder or a diagnostic artifact, partially related to higher sensitivity in detecting this condition, and partially related to overdiagnosis [34].

Elderly patients

As many as one in ten cases of bipolar disorder first present after the age of 50 years [62]. The lifetime prevalence of bipolar disorder in individuals over 65 is thought to range from 0.5% to 1%, and it is estimated that at least 8% to 10% of geriatric psychiatric admissions are for bipolar disorder [63,64].

Individuals who develop bipolar disorder in later life are less likely than others to have a family history of bipolar disorder and may also exhibit longer episode durations or more frequent episodes [65]. Around half of patients with onset of mania at older ages have had previous depressive episodes, often with a long latency period before the first manic episode [66].

As in younger patients, bipolar disorder in elderly people may also be associated with general medical conditions, medications, or substance use. In particular, the onset of mania in later life is associated with high rates of medical comorbidity, especially neurological diseases including right hemispherical cortical or subcortical lesions [66]. An accelerated age-related decrease in levels of brain-derived neurotrophic factor (BDNF), which is normally responsible for the development of long-term memory, has been seen in older patients with bipolar disorder [67].

References

1   World Health Organization (WHO). *The ICD-10 Classification of Mental and Behavioral Disorders: Clinical Description and Diagnostic Guidelines (CDDG-10)*. Geneva, Switzerland: WHO; 1992.

2   World Health Organization. *The ICD-10 Classification of Mental and Behavioral Disorders: Diagnostic Criteria for Research (DCR-10)*. Geneva, Switzerland: WHO; 1993.

3   American Psychiatric Association. *Diagnostic and Statistical Manual of Mental Disorders, 4th Edn, Text Revision (DSM-IV-TR)*. Washington DC: American Psychiatric Association; 2000.

4   First MB, Spitzer RL, Gibbon M, et al. *Structures Clinical Interview for DSM-IV Axis I Disorders – Clinician Version (SCID-IV)*. Washington DC: American Psychiatric Press; 1997.

5   Wing JK, Cooper JE, Sartorius N. *The Measurement and Classification of Psychiatric Symptoms*. 10th ed. London, UK: Cambridge University Press; 1998.

6   American Psychiatric Association. Practice guideline for the treatment of patients with bipolar disorder (revision). *Am J Psychiatry*. 2002;159(4 suppl):1-50.

7   Suppes T, Kelly DI, Perla JM. Challenges in the management of bipolar depression. *J Clin Psychiatry*. 2005;66(suppl 5):11-16.

8   Angst J, Gamma A, Bowden CL, et al. Diagnostic criteria for bipolarity based on an international sample of 5,635 patients with DSM-IV major depressive episodes. *Eur Arch Psychiatry Clin Neurosci*. 2012; 262:3-11.

9   Scottish Intercollegiate Guidelines Network (SIGN). *Guideline No.82: Bipolar Affective Disorder*. Edinburgh, UK: SIGN; 2005.

10 Fennig S, Kovasznay B, Rich C, et al. Six-month stability of psychiatric diagnoses in first-admission patients with psychosis. *Am J Psychiatry*. 1994;151:1200-1208.

11 Salvatore P, Baldessarini R, Tohen M, et al. McLean–Harvard International First-Episode Project: Two-year stability of DSM-IV diagnoses in 500 first-episode psychotic disorder patients. *J Clin Psychiatry*. 2009;70:458-466.

12 Hirschfeld RM, Lewis L, Vornik LA. Perceptions and impact of bipolar disorder: how far have we really come? Results of the National Depressive and Manic-Depressive Association 2000 survey of individuals with bipolar disorder. J Clin Psychiatry 2003; 64:161-174.

13 Bowden CL. Strategies to reduce misdiagnosis of bipolar depression. *Psychiatr Serv*. 2001;52:51-55.

14 Angst J, Azorin JM, Bowden CH, et al, the BRIDGE Study Group. Prevalence and characteristics of undiagnosed bipolar disorders in patients with a major depressive episode: the BRIDGE Study. *Arch Gen Psychiatry*. 2011;68:791-799.

15 Post RM, Leverich GS, Kupka R, et al. Early-onset bipolar disorder and treatment delay are risk factors for poor outcome in adulthood. *J Clin Psychiatry*. 2010;71:864-872.

16 Post RM. Transduction of psychosocial stress into the neurobiology of recurrent affective disorder. *Am J Psychiatry*. 1992;149:999-1010.

17 Swann AC, Bowden CL, Morris D, et al. Depression during mania. Treatment response to lithium or divalproex. *Arch Gen Psychiatry*. 1997;54:37-42.

18 Altshuler LL, Post RM, Leverich GS, et al. Antidepressant-induced mania and cycle acceleration: a controversy revisited. *Am J Psychiatry*. 1995;152:1130-1138.

19 Ghaemi SN, Boiman EE, Goodwin FK. Diagnosing bipolar disorder and the effect of antidepressants: a naturalistic study. *J Clin Psychiatry*. 2000;61:804-808.

20 Valentí M, Pacchiarotti I, Rosa AR, et al. Bipolar mixed episodes and antidepressants: a cohort study of bipolar I disorder patients. *Bipolar Disord*. 2011;13:145-154.

21 Goodwin GM, Anderson I, Arango C, et al. ECNP consensus meeting. Bipolar depression. Nice, March 2007. *Eur Neuropsychopharmacol*. 2008;18:535-549.

22 Swann AC, Bowden CL, Calabrese JR, et al. Differential effect of number of previous episodes of affective disorder on response to lithium or divalproex in acute mania. *Am J Psychiatry*. 1999;156:1264-1266.

23 Tondo L, Baldessarini RJ. Reduced suicide risk during lithium maintenance treatment. *J Clin Psychiatry*. 2000;61(suppl 9):97-104.

24 Pacchiarotti I, Valentí M, Colom F, et al. Differential outcome of bipolar patients receiving antidepressant monotherapy versus combination with an antimanic drug. *J Affect Disord*. 2011;129:321-326.

25 Geller B, Cooper TB, Sun K, et al. Double-blind and placebo-controlled study of lithium for adolescent bipolar disorders with secondary substance dependency. *J Am Acad Child Adolesc Psychiatry*. 1998;37:171-178.

26 Grande I, de Arce R, Jiménez-Arriero MÁ, et al. Patterns of pharmacological maintenance treatment in a community mental health services bipolar disorder cohort study (SIN-DEPRES). *Int J Neuropsychopharmacol*. 2012; epub ahead of print.

27 FDA Public Health Advisory. Worsening depression and suicidality in patients being treated with antidepressant medications. March 22, 2004. FDA website. www.fda.gov/cder/drug/antidepressants/AntidepressanstPHA.htm. Accessed September 17, 2012.

28 Food and Drug Administration (FDA). Antidepressant use in children, adolescents, and adults. May 2, 2007. FDA website. www.fda.gov/Drugs/DrugSafety/InformationbyDrugClass/ucm096273.htm. Accessed September 17, 2012.

29 Vieta E. Case for caution, case for action. *Bipolar Disord*. 2003;5:434-435.

30 Vieta E. Overcoming the current approach in bipolar disorder research: towards DSM-V and beyond. *J Psychopharmacol*. 2008;22:406-407.

31 Baldessarini RJ, Leahy L, Arcona S, et al. Patterns of psychotropic drug prescription for U.S. patients with diagnoses of bipolar disorders. *Psychiatr Serv*. 2007;58:85-91.

32 Vieta E. Role of antidepressants in bipolar depression. *J Clin Psychiatry*. 2010;71:e21.

33 Zimmerman M, Ruggero CJ, Chelminski I, et al. Is bipolar disorder overdiagnosed? *J Clin Psychiatry*. 2008;69:935-940.

34 Moreno C, Laje G, Blanco C, Jiang H, Schmidt AB, Olfson M. National trends in the outpatient diagnosis and treatment of bipolar disorder in youth. *Arch Gen Psychiatry*. 2007;64:1032-1039.

35 Skirrow C, Hosang GM, Farmer AE, et al. An update on the debated association between ADHD and bipolar disorder across the lifespan. *J Affect Disord*. 2012;141:143-159.

36 Yatham LN, Kennedy SH, O'Donovan C, et al. Canadian Network for Mood and Anxiety Treatments (CANMAT) guidelines for the management of patients with bipolar disorder: consensus and controversies. *Bipolar Disord*. 2005;7(suppl 3):5-69.

37 Vieta E. *Guide to Assessment Scales in Bipolar Disorder*. London, UK: Current Medicine Group; 2006.

38 Hirschfeld RMA, Williams JB, Spitzer RL, et al. Development and validation of a screening instrument for bipolar spectrum disorder: the Mood Disorder Questionnaire. *Am J Psychiatry*. 2000;157:1873-1875.

39 Zimmerman M. Misuse of the Mood Disorders Questionnaire as a case-finding measure and a critique of the concept of using a screening scale for bipolar disorder in psychiatric practice. *Bipolar Disord*. 2012;14:127-134.

40 Ghaemi SN, Miller CJ, Berv DA, et al. Sensitivity and specificity of a new bipolar spectrum diagnostic scale. *J Affect Disord*. 2005;84:273-277.

41 Beck AT, Ward CH, Mendelson M, et al. An inventory for measuring depression. *Arch Gen Psychiatry*. 1961; 4:561-571.

42 Montgomery SA, Asberg M. A new depression scale designed to be sensitive to change. *Br J Psychiatry*. 1979; 134:382-389.

43 Calabrese JR, Bowden CL, Sachs GS, et al. A double-blind placebo-controlled study of lamotrigine monotherapy in outpatients with bipolar I depression. Lamictal 602 Study Group. *J Clin Psychiatry*. 1999;60:79-88.

44 Hamilton M. A rating scale for depression. *J Neurol Neurosurg Psychiatry*. 1960;23:56-62.

45 Hamilton M. Rating depressive patients. *J Clin Psychiatry*. 1980;41:21-24.

46 Altman EG, Hedeker DR, Janicak PG, et al. The Clinician-Administered Rating Scale for Mania (CARS-M): development, reliability and validity. *Biol Psychiatry*. 1994;36:124-134.

47 Young RC, Biggs JT, Ziegler VT, et al. A rating scale for mania: reliability, validity and sensitivity. *Br J Psychiatry*. 1978;133:429-435.

48 Angst J, Adolfsson R, Benazzi F, et al. The HCL-32: towards a self-assessment tool for hypomanic symptoms in outpatients. *J Affect Disord*. 2005;88:217-233.

49 Vieta E, Sánchez-Moreno J, Bulbena A, et al; EDHIPO (Hypomania Detection Study) Group. Cross validation with the mood disorder questionnaire (MDQ) of an instrument for the detection of hypomania in Spanish: the 32 item hypomania symptom check list (HCL-32). *J Affect Disord*. 2007;101:43-55.

50 Chengappa KN, Kupfer DJ, Frank E, et al. Relationship of birth cohort and early age at onset of illness in a bipolar disorder case registry. *Am J Psychiatry*. 2003;160:1636-1642.

51 Lewinsohn PM, Klein DN, Seeley JR. Bipolar disorders in a community sample of older adolescents: prevalence, phenomenology, comorbidity, and course. *J Am Acad Child Adolesc Psychiatry*. 1995;34:454-463.

52 Rao U, Ryan N, Birmaher B et al. Unipolar depression in adolescents: clinical outcome in adulthood. *J Am Acad Child Adolesc Psychiatry*. 1995;34:566-578.

53 Perlis R, Miyahara S, Marangell L, et al. Long-term implications of early onset in bipolar disorder: data from the first 1000 participants in the systematic treatment enhancement program for bipolar disorder (STEP-BD). *Biol Psychiatry*. 2004;55:875-881.

54 Masi G, Toni C, Perugi G, et al. Anxiety disorders in children and adolescents with bipolar disorder: a neglected comorbidity. *Can J Psychiatry*. 2001;46:797-802.

55 State R, Frye M, Altshuler L, et al. Chart review of the impact of attention-deficit/hyperactivity disorder comorbidity on response to lithium or divalproex sodium in adolescent mania. *J Clin Psychiatry*. 2004;65:1057-1063.

56 Faedda G, Baldessarini R, Glovinsky I, et al. Pediatric bipolar disorder: phenomenology and course of illness. *Bipolar Disord*. 2004; 6:305-313.

57 Nolan TM, Bond L, Adler R, et al. Child Behaviour Checklist classification of behaviour disorder. *J Paediatr Child Health*. 1996;32:405-411.

58 Gracious BL, Youngstrom EA, Findling RL, et al. Discriminative validity of a parent version of the Young Mania Rating Scale. *J Am Acad Child Adolesc Psychiatry*. 2002;41:1350-1359.

59 Shaffer D, Gould MS, Brasic J, et al. A children's global assessment scale (CGAS). *Arch Gen Psychiatry*. 1983;40:1228-1231.

60 Geller B, Warner K, Williams M, et al. Prepubertal and young adolescent bipolarity versus ADHD: assessment and validity using the WASH-U-KSADS, CBCL and TRF. *J Affect Disord*. 1998;51:93-100.

61 Geller B, Zimerman B, Williams M, et al. Reliability of the Washington University in St Louis Kiddie Schedule for Affective Disorders and Schizophrenia (WASH-U-KSADS) mania and rapid cycling sections. *J Am Acad Child Adolesc Psychiatry*. 2001;40:450-455.

62 Sajatovic M. Treatment of bipolar disorder in older adults. *Int J Geriatr Psychiatry*. 2002;17:865-873.

63 Sajatovic M, Chen P. Geriatric bipolar disorders. *Psychiatr Clin North Am*. 2011;34:319-333.

64 Depp CA, Jeste DV. Bipolar disorder in older adults: a critical review. *Bipolar Disord*. 2004;6:343-367.

65 Young RC, Klerman GL. Mania in late life: focus on age at onset. *Am J Psychiatry*. 1992;149:867-876.

66 Shulman KI, Herrmann N. The nature and management of mania in old age. *Psychiatr Clin North Am*. 1999;22:649-665.

67 Yatham LN, Kapczinski F, Andreazza AC, et al. Accelerated age-related decrease in brain-derived neurotrophic factor levels in bipolar disorder. *Int J Neuropsychopharmacol*. 2009;12:137-139.

Chapter 5

Suicide risk

Patients with bipolar disorder are at extremely high risk for suicide. It is estimated that one-third to one-half of bipolar disorder patients attempt suicide at least once during their lifetime [1]. The risk of suicide may be greater in bipolar II than bipolar I disorder, in light of the greater preponderance of recurrent severe depression [2], although the rates of attempted suicide are similar [3].

In a meta-analysis of English language reports on the mortality of mental disorders, the overall rate of suicide among bipolar patients was estimated at 0.40% per year, versus an international population average of 0.017%. This equates to a standardized mortality ratio of 22, compared with around 20 in unipolar depression and 8.4 in schizophrenia [4,5]. The annual risk of suicide attempts is about 0.9%, which is 30- to 60-fold higher than the 0.015% rate seen in the general population [6].

Suicide attempts by patients with bipolar disorder have a very high risk of fatality. One in five suicide attempts by bipolar patients is completed, versus one in 10–20 in the general population [7]. Bipolar patients may attempt suicide earlier during the index episode than other psychiatric patients [8].

Assessing suicide risk in clinical practice

Several risk factors for suicide have been identified in bipolar disorder, and many are additive. They include a history of suicide attempts, a family history of suicidal behavior, a greater severity and number of

E. Vieta, *Managing Bipolar Disorder in Clinical Practice*,
DOI: 10.1007/978-1-908517-94-4_5, © Springer Healthcare 2013

depressive episodes, alcohol/substance abuse, pessimism, aggression/ impulsivity, pervasive insomnia, early traumatic events, and negative life experiences [9–13].

Early age of illness onset is a major risk factor for suicide. The longitudinal Course and Outcome of Bipolar Youth study found that 32% of patients who were diagnosed with bipolar disorder in childhood or adolescence had attempted suicide at least once during their lifetime, and 67% of that group had a history of moderate or severe suicidal ideation [14]. A 5-year follow-up of 413 patients from that study noted a suicide attempt rate of 18% during that time period. Attempters were more likely to be female and have had taken at least one antidepressant [15].

Among the phases of bipolar disorder, depressive episodes carry the highest suicide risk, followed by mixed states (particularly mixed depression), with episodes of mania having the lowest risk. Rapid cycling and axis I and II comorbidity are also major risk factors [1].

The risk factors for attempted suicide partially but not fully overlap with the risk factors for completed suicide, and include previous attempts, family history of suicide, psychiatric comorbidity (particularly substance abuse and personality disorders), depressive symptoms during index episode, rapid cycling, depressive predominant polarity, and some medications, including some antidepressants (in children) and anticonvulsants (in epilepsy) [16–24]. Factors that should be considered when assessing suicide risk in patients with bipolar disorder are summarized in Table 5.1 [1].

Strategies to reduce suicide risk

Judging suicidal risk is inherently imperfect; therefore, the risks and benefits of intervention must be carefully weighed and documented. As a rule, suicide risk is associated with depression, and risk assessment is always advisable during episodes of bipolar depression. Mixed, anxious episodes may also carry high risk. However, long-term strategies are also important to reduce suicide risk by preventing new episodes and reducing chronic subsyndromal symptoms.

Clinically relevant and explorable risk factors of suicidal behavior in bipolar disorder patients

Longitudinal risk factors	
Personality features	• Aggressive/impulsive personality traits • Cyclothymic temperament
Personal and/or family history	• Early negative life events (separation, emotional, physical, and sexual abuse) • Acute psychosocial stressors • Permanent adverse life situations • Family history of mood disorders in first- and second-degree relatives • Family history of suicide and/or suicide attempt in first- and second-degree relatives
Illness course	• Bipolar II diagnosis • Early onset • Early stage of the illness • Longer duration of untreated illness (delayed diagnosis or proper diagnosis) • Polarity of first episode • Predominantly depressive course • Number of previous episodes • Prior suicide attempt/ideation (especially violent/highly lethal methods) • Rapid cycling course
Cross-sectional risk factors	
Characteristics of current mood episode	• Severe major depressive episode • Agitated or mixed depressive mixed state • Dysphoric mania • Severe anxiety and insomnia • Current suicide attempt, plan, ideation • Hopelessness, guilt, few reasons for living • Psychotic features • Atypical features • Bipolar II diagnosis • Comorbid Axis I (anxiety disorder, substance-use disorders) and Axis II disorders • Serious medical illness • Lack of medical treatment • Lack of social or family support • Initiation and first few days of the treatment • First few weeks and months after hospital discharge

Table 5.1 Clinically relevant and explorable risk factors of suicidal behavior in bipolar disorder patients. Reproduced with permission from Gonda et al [1].

Pharmacotherapy

Suicide has never been the primary endpoint of a clinical trial because rates are too low to make such a trial feasible. However, evidence from observational studies indicates that suicide rates are lower in patients who receive long-term treatment [25]. Furthermore, lithium may have particular efficacy, despite its risk of toxicity and high lethality in overdose [26].

In a meta-analysis of 22 studies of patients with major affective illness (mainly bipolar disorder), the risk of completed suicide was 8.85 times lower with long-term lithium treatment than without it [27]. The rate of completed suicides was still 10 times higher than in the general population, however [28].

Another systematic review of 32 randomized trials in patients with mood disorders found that lithium treatment was effective in preventing suicide, deliberate self-harm, and death from all causes (Figure 5.1) [29]. The comparators in these trials included placebo, amitriptyline, carbamazepine, and lamotrigine. These findings were confirmed by a meta-analysis of six trials that directly compared lithium with anticonvulsants (valproate, carbamazepine, and lamotrigine). Suicide risk was 2.86 times greater with anticonvulsant therapy than with lithium [30]. Clozapine and perhaps other atypical antipsychotics might also have some antisuicidal effects, although it has not been specifically proven in bipolar illness [31].

Psychotherapy

The efficacy of other suicide prevention strategies, such as psychosocial treatments, is difficult to prove due to small sample sizes and patient selection bias. However, a study by Rucci et al offers support for the efficacy of pharmacotherapy and adjunctive psychotherapy [32]. In this study, 175 patients with bipolar I disorder were recruited during an acute mood episode and received lithium plus psychotherapy specific to bipolar disorder (including help in regularizing daily routines) or non-specific intensive clinical management involving regular visits with empathetic clinicians.

Compared with before study entry, suicide attempts were reduced three-fold during the acute treatment phase and 17.5-fold during maintenance treatment (Figure 5.2), and no patient who had attempted suicide before enrolment did so during the study period. The authors concluded that a treatment program in a 'maximally supporting clinical environment' can reduce suicidal behavior in high-risk bipolar patients [32].

The goal of psychotherapy should be to recognize the links between suicide and depression and to be aware of these 'warning signs'. Targets for psychosocial intervention could include not only depression and suicidal ideation, but also family issues, social rhythms, grief issues surrounding having bipolar disorder, and interpersonal deficits [33].

Patient and carer education
Educating patients and their carers about the risk of suicide in bipolar disorder is an important part of the long-term treatment plan. This may involve: discussing the importance of long-term treatments, particularly lithium, in lowering suicide risk; identifying early warning signs of relapse; teaching stress management techniques; and developing a plan of action should prodromal symptoms arise. Suicide must be discussed as an illness-related behavior. Psychological interventions to improve the long-term prognosis of bipolar disorder are discussed further in Chapter 10.

Forest plots showing meta-analyses of randomized trials comparing lithium with placebo or active comparators

Study	Numbers of suicides/patients			Weight (%)	Peto odds ratio (95% CI)
	Lithium	Comparator	Favors lithium ← → Favors comparator		
Suicide					
Lithium versus placebo					
Subtotal (95% CI)	0/146	2/143		15.7	0.13 (0.01–2.04)
Lithium versus amitriptyline					
Subtotal (95% CI)	0/97	2/91		15.7	0.13 (0.01–2.05)
Lithium versus carbamazepine					
Subtotal (95% CI)	2/139	6/146		61.4	0.37 (0.09–1.51)
Lithium versus lamotrigine					
Subtotal (95% CI)	0/121	1/221		7.2	0.21 (0.00–12.83)
Total (95% CI)	**2/503**	**11/601**		**100.0**	**0.26 (0.09–0.77)**
Suicide and self-harm					
Lithium versus placebo					
Subtotal (95% CI)	0/267	3/254		15.5	0.13 (0.03–1.25)
Lithium versus amitriptyline					
Subtotal (95% CI)	0/97	2/91		10.3	10.3 (0.03–2.05)
Lithium versus carbamazepine					
Subtotal (95% CI)	2/139	11/146		64.4	0.25 (0.08–0.76)
Lithium versus lamotrigine					
Subtotal (95% CI)	0/167	2/280		9.8	0.19 (0.03–3.24)
Total (95% CI)	**2/670**	**18/771**		**100.0**	**0.21 (0.06–0.50)**

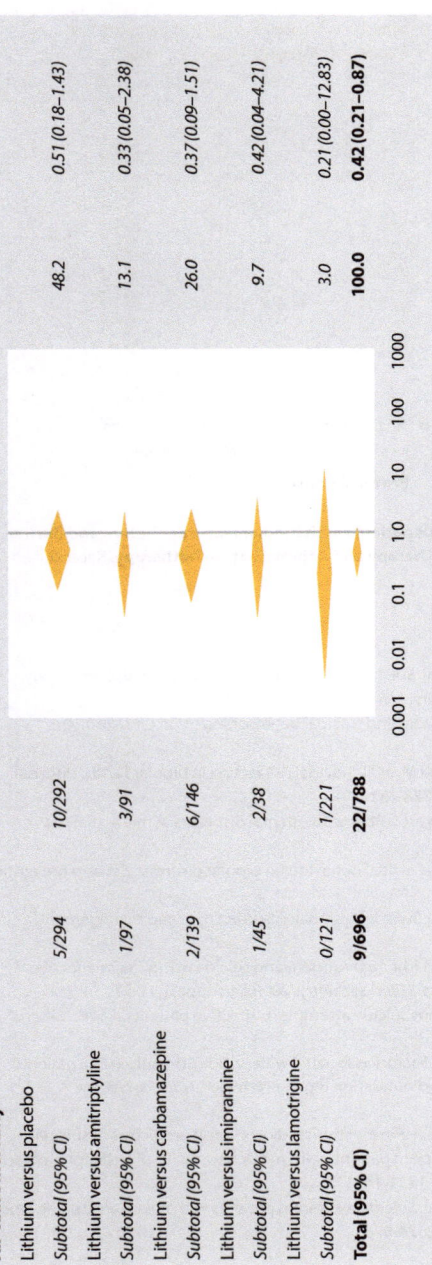

Figure 5.1 Forest plots showing meta-analyses of randomized trials comparing lithium with placebo or active comparators. CI, confidence interval. Adapted from Cipriani et al [29].

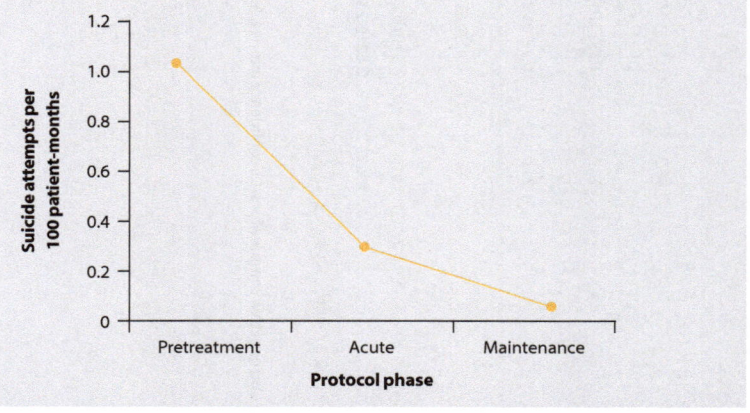

Rate of suicide attempts of patients with bipolar I disorder before and during intensive treatment with pharmacotherapy and adjunctive psychotherapy

Figure 5.2 Rate of suicide attempts of patients with bipolar I disorder before and during intensive treatment with pharmacotherapy and adjunctive psychotherapy. Reproduced from Rucci et al [25].

References

1   Gonda X, Pompili M, Serafini G, et al. Suicidal behavior in bipolar disorder: epidemiology, characteristics and major risk factors. *J Affect Disord*. 2012;143:16-26.
2   Rihmer Z, Pestality P. Bipolar II disorder and suicidal behavior. *Psychiatr Clin North Am*. 1999;22:667-673.
3   Undurraga J, Baldessarini RJ, Valenti M, et al. Suicidal risk factors in bipolar I and II disorder patients. *J Clin Psychiatry*. 2012;73:778-782.
4   Harris EC, Barraclough B. Suicide as an outcome for mental disorders. A meta-analysis. *Br J Psychiatry*. 1997;170:205-228.
5   Tondo L, Isacsson G, Baldessarini R. Suicidal behaviour in bipolar disorder: risk and prevention. *CNS Drugs*.2003;17:491-511.
6   Baldessarini RJ, Pompili M, Tondo L. Suicide in bipolar disorder: risks and management. *CNS Spectr*. 2006;11:465-471.
7   Baldessarini RJ, Tondo L, Hennen J. Lithium treatment and suicide risk in major affective disorders: update and new findings. *J Clin Psychiatry*. 2003;64(suppl 5):44-52.
8   Vieta E, Nieto E, Gasto C, et al. Serious suicide attempts in affective patients. *J Affect Disord*. 1992;24:147-152.
9   Leverich G, Altshuler L, Frye M, et al. Factors associated with suicide attempts in 648 patients with bipolar disorder in the Stanley Foundation Bipolar Network. *J Clin Psychiatry*. 2003;64:506-515.
10 Oquendo M, Galfalvy H, Russo S, et al. Prospective study of clinical predictors of suicidal acts after a major depressive episode in patients with major depressive disorder or bipolar disorder. *Am J Psychiatry*. 2004;161:1433-1441.
11 Strakowski S, McElroy S, Keck P, et al. Suicidality among patients with mixed and manic bipolar disorder. *Am J Psychiatry*. 1996;153:674-676.

12 Slama F, Bellivier F, Henry C, et al. Bipolar patients with suicidal behavior: toward the identification of a clinical subgroup. *J Clin Psychiatry*. 2004;65:1035-1039.

13 Dalton EJ, Cate-Carter TD, Mundo E, et al. Suicide risk in bipolar patients: the role of co-morbid substance use disorders. *Bipolar Disord*. 2003;5:58-61.

14 Goldstein TR, Birmaher B, Alexson D, et al. History of suicide attempts in pediatric bipolar disorder: factors associated with increased risk. *Bipolar Disord*. 2005;7:525-535.

15 Goldstein TR, Ha W, Axelson DA, et al. Predictors of prospectively examined suicide attempts among youth with bipolar disorder. *Arch Gen Psychiatry*. 2012; [epub ahead of print].

16 Romero S, Colom F, Iosif AM, et al. Relevance of family history of suicide in the long-term outcome of bipolar disorders. *J Clin Psychiatry*. 2007;68:1517-1521.

17 González-Pinto A, Aldama A, González C, et al. Predictors of suicide in first-episode affective and nonaffective psychotic inpatients: five-year follow-up of patients from a catchment area in Vitoria, Spain. *J Clin Psychiatry*. 2007;68:242-247.

18 Vieta E, Colom F, Corbella B, et al. Clinical correlates of psychiatric comorbidity in bipolar I patients. *Bipolar Disord*. 2001;3:253-258.

19 Vieta E, Colom F, Martínez-Arán A, et al. Bipolar II disorder and comorbidity. *Compr Psychiatry*. 2000;41:339-343.

20 Gonzalez-Pinto A, Mosquera F, Alonso M, et al. Suicidal risk in bipolar I disorder patients and adherence to long-term lithium treatment. *Bipolar Disord*. 2006;8:18-24.

21 Colom F, Vieta E, Daban C, et al. Clinical and therapeutic implications of predominant polarity in bipolar disorder. *J Affect Disord*. 2006;93:13-17.

22 Rosa AR, Andreazza AC, Kunz M, et al. Predominant polarity in bipolar disorder: diagnostic implications. *J Affect Disord*. 2008;107:45-51.

23 Cruz N, Vieta E, Comes M, et al; the EMBLEM Advisory Board. Rapid-cycling bipolar I disorder: Course and treatment outcome of a large sample across Europe. *J Psychiatr Res*. 2008;42:1068-1075.

24 Bridge JA, Iyengar S, Salary CB, et al. Clinical response and risk for reported suicidal ideation and suicide attempts in pediatric antidepressant treatment: a meta-analysis of randomized controlled trials. *JAMA*. 2007;297:1683-1696.

25 Angst F, Stassen HH, Clayton PJ, et al. Mortality of patients with mood disorders: follow-up over 34–38 years. *J Affect Disord*. 2002;68:167-181.

26 Fountoulakis KN, Vieta E, Bouras C, et al. A systematic review of existing data on long-term lithium therapy: neuroprotective or neurotoxic? *Int J Neuropsychopharmacol*. 2008;11:269-287.

27 Tondo L, Hennen J, Baldessarini RJ. Lower suicide risk with long-term lithium treatment in major affective illness: a meta-analysis. *Acta Psychiatr Scand*. 2001;104:163-172.

28 Baldessarini RJ, Tondo L, Hennen J. Treating the suicidal patient with bipolar disorder. Reducing suicide risk with lithium. *Ann NY Acad Sci*. 2001;932:24-38.

29 Cipriani A, Pretty H, Hawton K, et al. Lithium in the prevention of suicidal behavior and all-cause mortality in patients with mood disorders: a systematic review of randomized trials. *Am J Psychiatry*. 2005;162:1805-1819.

30 Baldessarini RJ, Tondo L. Suicidal risks during treatment of bipolar disorder patients with lithium versus anticonvulsants. *Pharmacopsychiatry*. 2009;42:72-75.

31 Tiihonen J, Wahlbeck K, Lönnqvist J, et al. Effectiveness of antipsychotic treatments in a nationwide cohort of patients in community care after first hospitalisation due to schizophrenia and schizoaffective disorder: observational follow-up study. *BMJ*. 2006;333:224.

32 Rucci P, Frank E, Kostelnik B, et al. Suicide attempts in patients with bipolar I disorder during acute and maintenance phases of intensive treatment with pharmacotherapy and adjunctive psychotherapy. *Am J Psychiatry*. 2002;159:1160-1164.

33 Fountoulakis KN, Gonda X, Siamouli M, et al. Psychotherapeutic intervention and suicide risk reduction in bipolar disorder: a review of the evidence. *J Affect Disord*. 2009;113:21-29.

Chapter 6

Overview of management options

Treatment principles and guidelines

Bipolar disorder is a chronic recurrent illness that requires a comprehensive and long-term program of medical care to help patients overcome the symptoms and functional impairment associated with the condition. A number of evidence-based practice guidelines are available to guide healthcare providers in the management of the disorder. Key treatment principles, as outlined in selected guidelines, are summarized below.

American Psychiatric Association [1]

Guideline title: Practice Guideline for the Treatment of Patients with Bipolar Disorder.

Date: 2nd edition, April 2002.

Key treatment principles:

- Although there is no cure for bipolar disorder, treatment can decrease the associated morbidity and mortality.
- Initial treatment of bipolar disorder requires a thorough assessment of the patient, with particular attention to the safety of the patient and those around him or her, as well as attention to possible comorbid psychiatric or medical illnesses.
- In addition to the current mood state, the clinician needs to consider the longitudinal history of the patient's illness.
- The primary treatment goal is to assess the patient's safety and level of functioning to decide the optimum treatment setting.

E. Vieta, *Managing Bipolar Disorder in Clinical Practice*, 73
DOI: 10.1007/978-1-908517-94-4_6, © Springer Healthcare 2013

- Subsequent goals include establishing and maintaining a therapeutic alliance, monitoring the patient's psychiatric status and response to treatment, providing education about bipolar disorder to the patient and their family, enhancing treatment compliance, promoting regular patterns of activity and sleep, anticipating stressors, identifying new episodes early, and minimizing functional impairments.
- Treatment recommendations are divided into the following categories: psychiatric management; acute treatment (manic or mixed episodes, depressive episodes, rapid cycling); and maintenance treatment.

Canadian Network for Mood and Anxiety Treatments [2]

Guideline title: Guidelines for the Management of Patients with Bipolar Disorder: Consensus and Controversies.

Date: 2nd edition, November 2005. Updates from 2007 and 2009 are available [3,4].

Key treatment principles:

- As patients require a long-term, multidisciplinary management plan, the Chronic Disease Management Model should be applied (Table 6.1).
- The first step is stabilization of the acute episode (especially patients in the manic/hypomanic phase), including determining whether patients are a danger to themselves or others.
- After initial pharmacotherapy and related clinical management, care should ideally be provided by a healthcare team that includes at least one other health professional in addition to the physician, typically a nurse who may provide detailed psychoeducation, additional monitoring, and support.

- The third step involves the provision of robust psychoeducation, which would include preparing the patient to become actively involved in self-management, identifying ways to collaborate most effectively with health providers, teaching key facts about bipolar disorder, teaching recognition of early signs of relapse, identifying a relapse drill, and learning a variety of key stress management techniques, including careful attention to sleep regulation and avoidance of substance misuse; family and key friends should be involved in part of the psychoeducation.
- Psychosocial treatments should be tailored to the specific needs of the patient; the patient should be connected to other community resources to enhance support and autonomy.

British Association for Psychopharmacology [5]

Guideline title: Evidence-Based Guidelines for Treating Bipolar Disorder.
Date: 2nd edition, June 2009.
Key treatment principles:
- The fundamentals for patients are diagnosis, access to services, the safety of patients and others, and enhanced care.
- Enhanced care comprises the following principles: establishing and maintaining a therapeutic alliance; educating yourself and then the patient and his or her family about the disorder; enhancing treatment adherence; promoting awareness of stressors, sleep disturbance, and early signs of relapse, and regular patterns of activity; evaluating and managing functional impairments; and increasing the focus of care planning in women of childbearing age.
- Specific treatment recommendations are divided into the following categories: acute manic or mixed episodes; acute depressive episodes; long-term treatment; treatment in special situations (eg, elderly, women of childbearing age); and physical health.

The Chronic Disease Management Model: elements of a healthcare system for effective care of patients with chronic disorders

Self-management support

- Empower and prepare patients to manage their health and healthcare
- Use effective self-management support strategies that include assessment, goal setting, action planning, problem solving, and follow-up

Decision support

- Promote clinical care that is consistent with scientific evidence and patient preferences
- Embed evidence-based guidelines into daily clinical practice and share this and other information with patients to encourage their participation
- Use proven provider education methods

Community

- Encourage patients to participate in effective community programs
- Form partnerships with community organizations

Delivery system design

- Provide clinical care and self-management support that patients understand and that fits with their cultural background
- Ensure regular follow-up by the care team, with defined tasks for different team members
- Provide clinical case management services for complex patients

Clinical information systems

- Provide timely reminders for providers and patients
- Facilitate individual patient care planning
- Share information with patients and providers to coordinate care

Health system

- Measure outcomes and use information to promote effective improvement strategies aimed at comprehensive system change
- Develop agreements that facilitate care coordination within and across organizations

Table 6.1 The Chronic Disease Management Model: Elements of a healthcare system for effective care of patients with chronic disorders. Reproduced with permission from Yatham et al [2].

World Federation of Societies of Biological Psychiatry [7–9]

Guideline title: The WFSBP guidelines for the biological treatment of bipolar disorders. This guideline does not include general principles of treatment and is focused on the biological treatment of depression, mania, and maintenance. The depression guidelines were updated in 2009 and the mania guidelines were updated in 2010.

Goals of intervention

The goals of intervention differ according to the phase of illness and the prevailing mood state. In the acute phase, treatment is aimed at stabilizing the current mood episode with the goal of achieving remission, defined as a complete return to baseline level of functioning and a virtual lack of symptoms. In the maintenance phase, the goal of treatment is to optimize protection against recurrence of depressive, mixed, manic, or hypomanic episodes. At the same time, attention should be devoted to maximizing patient functioning and minimizing subthreshold symptoms and adverse effects of treatment. The goals of intervention in bipolar disorder are summarized in Table 6.2.

Producing a treatment plan

Given the recurrent, chronic nature of bipolar disorder, a long-term preventive strategy that combines medication and psychosocial treatments is optimal for managing the disorder over time. Strategies that underpin the production of a treatment plan include weighing evidence, clinical assessment, education, negotiation, intervention, and multidisciplinary collaboration.

Despite the proliferation of treatment algorithms and guidelines, managing bipolar disorder challenges even the most experienced clinician. Numerous factors can complicate clinical management, and include:

- variability in symptoms and disease course;
- unreliability of the patient's self-assessment;
- high rates of comorbid substance abuse, anxiety disorders, and medical illness;
- substantial risk of suicide and other potentially severe adverse outcomes;
- need for polypharmacy, increasing the risk of side effects and non-compliance;
- poor understanding of bipolar disorder among family and friends; and
- lack of evidence to guide treatment strategies in children and elderly people.

The decalog of goals of intervention in bipolar disorder

1. To ensure the safety of the patient and others
2. To treat and reduce the severity of acute mood episodes when they occur
3. To treat psychotic symptoms when they occur
4. To avoid cycling from one episode to another
5. To prevent suicidal behavior
6. To reduce the frequency of mood episodes
7. To treat subthreshold symptoms
8. To treat comorbidities and cognitive problems
9. To increase the patient's and caregiver's knowledge about the disorder and enhance treatment adherence
10. To help the patient function as effectively as possible between episodes

Table 6.2 The decalog of goals of intervention in bipolar disorder.

Treatment options for bipolar disorder are extremely varied, and the targets and methods of intervention need to be individualized to meet the unique circumstances of each patient. In particular, it is necessary to determine – based on the patient's current diagnosis, symptom profile, and past history – whether priority should be given to tolerability or efficacy. Treatment can then be organized around the strategy that best serves the current priority. A sequential care strategy gives the highest priority to tolerability, whereas an urgent care strategy gives highest priority to immediate efficacy. As with other medical conditions, risk assessment drives the treatment priorities.

Assessment and treatment issues

Duration and phases of treatment

The complex task of treatment planning can be streamlined by considering the changing needs of patients during the acute, continuation, and discontinuation/maintenance phases of treatment (Figure 6.1) [10].

Acute treatment is used from the beginning of a manic or depressive episode (or as soon as the clinician is aware of the episode) until remission with the aim of improving overt clinical symptoms. Each individual trial of acute treatment is carried out to one of three endpoints:

1. discontinuation due to adverse effects;
2. discontinuation due to lack of response; and
3. successful resolution of the acute episode.

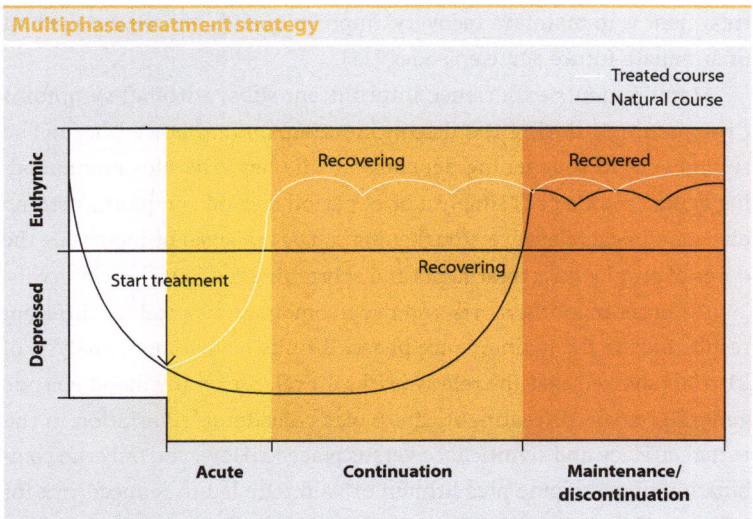

Multiphase treatment strategy

Figure 6.1 Multiphase treatment strategy. Reproduced from Sachs [10].

Common problems during the acute phase include treatment intolerance, inadequate dosage, partial response, and non-response.

A clinical status of 'recovering' indicates remission of acute symptoms and defines the continuation phase of treatment. The length of this phase is based on the clinician's estimate of the point at which spontaneous remission would have occurred had the patient not been treated. Thus, the duration of continuation treatment is determined by the natural course of illness, and aims to deal with ongoing vulnerability, even in the absence of overt symptoms. The most frequently encountered problem is relapse with return of full syndromal or continued symptomatic status. Successful acute therapies are therefore continued at full dosage for a period of time to reduce the risk of relapse.

The maintenance or discontinuation phase begins when the patient is declared to have recovered from the acute episode. Initially the aim is to monitor for recurrence while gradually tapering medication, and may involve medications used in the acute phase becoming part of the long-term maintenance regimen. Ultimately, the goal of maintenance treatment is to maintain recovery, improve quality of life, and prevent or attenuate future acute episodes [11].

Many patients experience intermittent subsyndromal symptoms ('roughening') during the discontinuation/maintenance phase. The significance of roughening depends on whether it heralds an impending acute episode or is simply a brief period of mild symptoms with no obvious clinical relevance. Roughening can be managed by increasing the doses of prophylactic treatments and shortening the follow-up intervals.

Different monotherapies and drug combinations produce different results during the maintenance phase. Results from a meta-analysis of 21 trials showed that the relative risks for relapse of any mood episode generally favored treatment; there was considerable variation in the actual efficacy and significance versus placebo. However, only the combination of quetiapine plus lithium or valproate led to reduced risk for relapse of manic/mixed and depressive episodes [12].

There is considerable debate about the optimal duration of maintenance therapy, particularly after a depressive episode. As bipolar disorder is currently recognized as a chronic, recurring, and disabling condition, most experts advise long-term maintenance therapy right from the first episode.

Treatment response

Most first-line treatments for an acute bipolar mood episode can be expected to produce an appreciable clinical effect within 10–14 days. If symptoms remain uncontrolled after this time, the first step should be to optimize the dose of current medication and to ensure that blood levels are in the therapeutic range. It is also important to identify issues of non-compliance with medication, which is a frequent cause of episode recurrence.

If symptoms continue unabated, further options include adding on or switching to a second or third agent, again ensuring optimal dosing and compliance. It is recommended that each pharmacotherapeutic regimen be tried for at least 2 weeks before concluding that the patient is unlikely to respond (usually defined as <30% reduction in symptoms), but in clinical practice the pressure to discharge an inpatient or the need to quickly ameliorate an outpatient generally require a faster turn-around of medication unless significant improvement is achieved. In patients with severe or treatment-resistant illness, electroconvulsive therapy (ECT) and novel or experimental treatments may be considered. In addition, there is some, but still limited, evidence that adjunctive psychological approaches can help augment the response to pharmacological therapy in acute episodes [13,14].

When selecting the primary treatment, the general rule is to use whatever was successful in treating the index episode. However, many patients will have breakthrough episodes regardless of their primary treatment. These patients will require combination therapy, and the best strategy is to start with the most established medications, moving to less proven agents if established treatments are ineffective or not tolerated. Table 6.3 lists the circumstances in which non-standard treatments may be appropriate; care should be taken to document the indication in the medical record [10].

Predominant polarity

The concept of predominant polarity may be relevant for the choice of long-term treatment of bipolar disorder [15,16], as shown in Table 6.4 [15]. Patients with at least two-thirds of their total number of episodes with a particular polarity (manic or depressive) may have defined typologies and treatment response. The majority of treatments, including psychosocial therapies [17], are more effective for one pole of the disorder than the other, with perhaps the only exception of quetiapine [18].

Indications for non-standard treatment	
Indication	**Example**
Standard treatments have failed	Use of stimulant after non-response to more than one standard antidepressants
Standard treatments are intolerable	Use of DHEA in patient with a history of severe headache during prior treatment with multiple standard agents with different mechanisms/structure
Innovative treatment compatible with standard treatment	Patient requests adjunctive use of omega-3 fatty acids
Standard treatments are unacceptable	Patient refuses standard treatments because of fears based on knowledge of individuals with unfavorable outcome

Table 6.3 Indications for non-standard treatment. DHEA, dehydroepiandrosterone. Reproduced from Sachs [10].

Predominant polarity typologies	
Depressive polarity	**Manic polarity**
• 60% bipolar disorder patients	• 40% bipolar disorder patients
• More bipolar II disorder	• More bipolar I disorder
• More depressive onset	• More manic onset
• More seasonal pattern	• Younger and earlier onset
• More suicide attempts	• More substance misuse
• Better long-term response to lamotrigine	• Better long-term response to atypical antipsychotics
• More antidepressant use	

Table 6.4 Predominant polarity typologies. Reproduced from Colom et al [15].

Patient monitoring

At each follow-up visit, the patient's clinical status should be determined and recorded in a systematic manner (Table 6.5) [10]. In view of time constraints, it can be very helpful if patients complete a self-report form in the waiting room, as well as daily mood charts that they bring to the consultation. Active patient collaboration with routine assessment not only increases the time available for more unstructured talk but also improves rapport by providing documentation of the patient's subjective experience.

The clinician can also benefit from using graphical charting, since knowledge of an individual patient's disease course is perhaps the most useful guide to planning treatment. The use of graphical mood charts greatly enhances the clinician's ability to quickly recognize patterns of illness and the impact of treatment. Over time, the mood chart data facilitate tracking of response to interventions, typical precipitants and prodromes, cycle frequency, patterns of illness, predominant polarity, and duration of episodes.

Compliance

Patients with bipolar disorder are frequently ambivalent about treatment, and it is estimated that one in three patients fails to take at least 30% of their prescribed medication [19]. Unfortunately, treatment non-adherence is an important cause of disease recurrence, as well as being associated with higher rates of both hospitalization and suicide [20–22]. In addition, non-adherence has been linked with a heightened severity of mood episodes [23].

	DSM-IV	Clinical status
Definitions for assignment of clinical status		
Fully syndromal	Depression Mania Hypomania Mixed	Depression Mania Hypomania Mixed
Subsyndromal	Partial recovery Symptoms subthreshold for full episode or <8 weeks with minimal symptoms	Continued symptomatic ≥3 moderate symptoms
Well	Recovered	Recovering ≤2 moderate symptoms Recovered >8 weeks with ≤2 moderate symptoms
New subsyndromal	–	Roughening >3 moderate symptoms following after meeting criteria for recovered

Table 6.5 Definitions for assignment of clinical status. Reproduced from Sachs [10].

There are many explanations for the high rates of non-adherence with treatment among bipolar disorder patients (Table 6.6 and Figure 6.2) [24,25]. Patients frequently lack insight, especially during a manic episode, and may not believe that they have a serious illness. They may also minimize or deny the reality of a previous episode or their own behavior and its consequences.

Another important factor for some patients is their reluctance to give up the experience of hypomania or mania. Patients often recall the increased energy, euphoria, heightened self-esteem, and ability to focus as very desirable and enjoyable, while minimizing or denying the subsequent devastating features of full-blown mania or the extended demoralization of a depressive episode.

Medication side effects, as well as costs and other demands, are a further consideration and should be minimized by all possible means. These include dose adjustments, once-daily administration, and switching between formulations [26]. Other efforts to improve compliance include user-friendly packaging, monitoring of pill taking, and even delivery of supplies of medicine. However, the psychological burden of needing long-term medication as such is also important [27]; results of a survey summarizing the main concerns of patients about drug treatment are shown in Figure 6.3 [28].

Factors influencing treatment adherence	
Negative factors	**Positive factors**
Younger age	Older age
Early onset	Marriage
History of non-adherence	High level of education
History of grandiosity	Treatment alliance
Mood-incongruent psychotic features	Social support
More hospitalizations or more previous episodes versus fewer episodes	Favorable influence by ideas of others
Male gender	Realize threat of illness and/or benefits of treatment
First year of treatment versus longer-duration prescribed medications	Recognition of adverse consequences of illness (eg, hospitalization)
Elevated mood, hypomania, mania, hyperthymia	External locus of control or dependence
Personality	
Comorbid drug/alcohol abuse	
Temperament (eg, sensation seeking)	
Cognitive deficits	
Anxiety regarding long-term safety of treatment/fear of side effects	
Denial of severity of illness; denial of need/poor insight	
Idea that moods controlled by medication/need more control; dislike dependence on meds	
Idea that taking medication reminded them that they had a chronic illness; stigma of 'chronic mental patient'	
Medication does not help depression	
Hassles of medication regimen	
'Missing highs'; especially in women	
Actual side effects	

Table 6.6 Factors influencing treatment adherence. Reproduced from Berk et al [24].

Several methods are used to enhance adherence with treatment. Effective interventions tend to involve the patient and family members, incorporate a good understanding of the disorder, medications, and related side effects, and be integrated into the long-term treatment plan [14]. Psychological interventions such as cognitive–behavioral therapy and psychoeducation are particularly effective, and these are discussed below and in Chapter 10.

Suicide risk

As discussed in Chapter 5, patients with bipolar disorder are at extremely high risk for suicide, with half of patients making at least one suicide

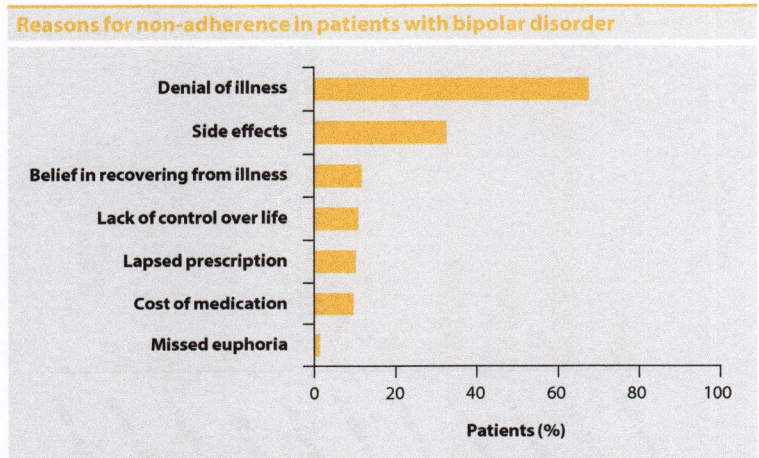

Figure 6.2 Reasons for non-adherence in patients with bipolar disorder. Patients may have cited more than one reason for non-adherence. Data taken from Keck et al [25].

attempt during their lifetime. Although the high rates of suicidal behavior associated with bipolar disorder may be greatly reduced by treatment, the clinical need for assessment and management of suicide risk remains constant.

In the absence of means to predict suicide accurately, clinicians must manage the risk through systematic assessment and by establishing suicide prevention as a key objective in the treatment plan. The initiation of treatment provides a good opportunity for integrating suicide prevention strategies into the general management strategy, when the discussion between clinician and patient should include suicidality as a potential and therefore expectable symptom of the disease. An initial individualized plan can be based on a review of current and lifetime risk factors, and may draw on interventions such as those summarized in Table 6.7 [10].

Suicide prevention strategies should be integrated into all phases of treatment. Prioritising patient needs separately during the acute, continuation, and maintenance phases of treatment adds clarity to the complex task of treatment planning (Table 6.8) [9]. For example, during the acute phase, the priorities are safety and amelioration of acute symptoms that frequently include suicidal ideation. In the early part of

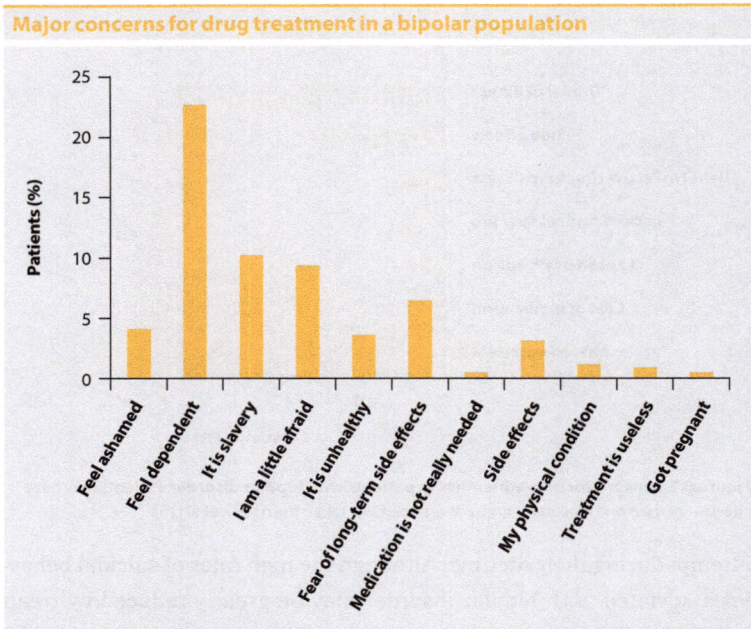

Major concerns for drug treatment in a bipolar population

Figure 6.3 Major concerns for drug treatment in a bipolar population. Reproduced from Vieta et al [28].

the continuation phase, clinical improvement can potentially heighten the risk of suicide by restoring energy and motivation to an otherwise suicidally depressed patient. Premature return to work or school may expose the patient to additional demoralizing stressors.

Finally, when the indicators of suicidal inclination diminish, risk-reduction strategies can be gradually tapered. During the maintenance phase, the risk of self-harm may be reduced by incorporating strategies for recognition and management into the treatment plan; in this context, suicide is discussed as a symptom of the disease rather than a trait of the individual patient.

Antidepressant discontinuation syndrome

Antidepressants have very limited efficacy in bipolar depression [29], but for many reasons most patients end up on antidepressants [30,31]. Treatment guidelines generally recommend that antidepressants be discontinued within 6 months of remission of depressive symptoms, with the rationale that continued antidepressant use might induce switches into mania or rapid cycling. As mentioned in Chapter 4, patients with bipolar I disorder treated with antidepressants who had mixed episodes during follow-up had higher switch rates and relapse rates than patients who had not had a mixed episode [32]. However, it is also possible that antidepressant discontinuation itself can precipitate a switch to acute hypomania or mania or a depressive relapse [33]. Given the paucity of evidence surrounding this issue, close monitoring is warranted at the time of antidepressant tapering/withdrawal. This may apply to the majority of treatment modalities in bipolar disorder: there may be an extremely delicate balance that, once achieved, can easily be lost by sudden treatment changes; but excessive polypharmacy should also be

Interventions to reduce risk
Non-specific interventions
To reduce inclination
Sustain therapeutic relationships
Sustain periods of wellness
Abstain from alcohol and unprescribed use of mood-altering substances
Treat substance abuse
Create a treatment contract with doctors and significant others, to empower them in high-risk situations
Keep a daily mood chart
Develop a list of triggers to depressive episodes
List 25 pleasurable activities and choose at least one each day
Maintain contact with treating doctors
Assess suicidal ideation at each clinical visit
Allow time for recovery before returning to work or school
Tell people ahead of time not to take offense to provocative statements
Ask supports not to ask you to do things that will be more of a burden on you
Plan future-oriented activities
To minimize opportunity
Restrict access to firearms
Minimize access to lethal means
Educate significant others to risk of suicide
Encourage social contact

Table 6.7 Interventions to reduce risk (continues overleaf).

Interventions to reduce risk (continued)	
Specific interventions	
To reduce inclination	
Treat acute episodes (specifically depression)	Sustain periods of wellness
Minimize time spent in isolation	Increase social contacts
Assess suicidal ideation at each clinic visit	Activate treatment contract
Maintain adherence to medication treatment	Attend AA/NA meetings
Keep patient's home alcohol and drug free	Participate in religious affiliation
Maintain good sleep hygiene and regular schedule	Maintain good personal hygiene
Consider psychotherapy	Learn a thought-stopping technique
Keep a journal	Limit caffeine intake
Implement problem-solving and coping skills	Exercise
To minimize opportunity	
Remove firearms, toxins, drugs	
Eliminate stockpile of potential toxins (drugs)	
Educate significant others to current risk of suicide	
Encourage social contact	
Minimize time spent in isolation	
Include a contingency plan for responding to missed appointments	
Include a contingency plan to manage decisions to end therapeutic relationships	
Consider hospitalization	

Table 6.7 Interventions to reduce risk (continued). AA, Alcoholics Anonymous; NA, Narcotics Anonymous. Reproduced from Sachs [10].

avoided, so it is advised to taper down the medications that need to be withdrawn in a progressive, but effective, way.

Psychotherapy

Although pharmacotherapy is the mainstay of treatment for bipolar disorder, the evidence base supporting psychosocial interventions has recently expanded. Combining pharmacotherapy with specific, tailored, psychosocial interventions can decrease the risk of relapse, improve treatment adherence, and reduce the number and length of hospitalizations. A multidisciplinary approach may also enhance long-term patient outcomes such as mood stability, occupational and social functioning, and overall quality of life [34]. The different but complementary goals of pharmacotherapy and psychotherapy for bipolar disorder are outlined in Table 6.9 [23].

Integration of suicide prevention strategies into the multiphase treatment plan

Phase	General	Suicide prevention
New patient intake	Education to understand bipolar illness and treatment options	Discuss bipolar illness as a suicide risk factor and need to manage risk
	Determine diagnosis: • current clinical status • lifetime diagnosis • comorbid conditions	Assess other risk and protective factors
		Include suicide prevention module in collaborative care plan
	Implement initial treatment plan	Determine need to immediate specific intervention
	Develop collaborative care plan	
	Encourage support building	
All follow-up visits	Determine current clinical status	Assess potential suicidality. Monitor inclination and opportunity
	Monitor: • stressors • comorbid conditions • psychoactive substance use • treatment response • adverse effects • adherence/concordance	Determine need to immediate specific intervention
	Determine follow-up interval	
Acute episode	Treatment for depression/mania	Assure safety: • review current personal risk factors • review/activate personal protective factors • choose venue adequate for management of current inclination and opportunity • dispense medications in safe quantity • determine need to alert supports • determine follow-up interval
	Implement harm reduction strategies as per collaborative care plan	
Continuation phase	Continue acute treatment strategies	Continue acute treatment strategies
		Monitor inclination and opportunity
Maintenance phase	Revise collaborative care plan	Consider revision of suicide prevention strategies: • pharmacological • support building • formal psychotherapies
	Implement prophylactic strategies: • monitor for impending episodes • manage adverse effects	

Table 6.8 Integration of suicide prevention strategies into the multiphase treatment plan.
Reproduced from Sachs [10].

However, psychosocial interventions are not useful for all patients, and are probably best used as adjuncts to medication for prophylaxis and during periods of remission to reduce the risk of further episodes. Psychosocial treatments with the greatest supportive evidence are

Goals of pharmacotherapy and psychotherapy for bipolar disorder
Goals of pharmacotherapy
To reduce inclination
• Treatment of acute episodes   • Treatment of psychotic episodes
Goals of combined pharmacotherapy and psychotherapy
• Prophylaxis of recurrences   • Treatment of anxiety and insomnia   • Prevention of suicide   • Avoiding drug abuse   • Treatment adherence   • Improving impairment
Goals of psychotherapy
• Information about and adjustment to chronic illness   • Improve interepisodic functioning   • Emotional support   • Family support   • Early identification of prodromal symptoms   • Coping with psychosocial consequences of past and future episodes

Table 6.9 Goals of pharmacotherapy and psychotherapy for bipolar disorder. Reproduced from Vieta [23].

psychoeducation, cognitive–behavioral therapy, interpersonal and social-rhythm therapy, and family-focused therapy (FFT), and these are discussed in more detail in Chapter 10.

Electroconvulsive therapy

Although controlled data are lacking, open studies and clinical experience suggest that ECT is effective in the treatment of acute bipolar mood episodes, including mania, depression (particularly with psychotic or catatonic features), and mixed states. Like pharmacological therapies for bipolar depression, ECT may induce switching into mania, but the switch can be treated with further ECT sessions anyway [35]. Given the relatively weak evidence base, ECT is recommended only after trials of adequate pharmacological therapies have failed. In addition, ECT is a potential treatment for severe mood episodes during pregnancy, and for patients who express a preference for ECT after discussion with the clinician. Maintenance sessions of ECT may also be considered for patients whose acute episode responded to ECT. The management of treatment-resistant bipolar disorder is discussed in more detail in Chapter 9.

Pharmacological options

An array of pharmacological agents is used in the acute and maintenance phases of bipolar disorder, and the evidence supporting different approaches is reviewed in a number of clinical guidelines issued by specialist groups (Table 6.10) [36].

Many of the recommendations for specific agents are supported by evidence from meta-analyses and/or randomized controlled clinical trials. The foundation of the treatment should be mood stabilisers, but there is little consensus on what is a mood stabiliser and which drugs would qualify for that definition. In general, however, a mood stabiliser is expected to have long-term efficacy in bipolar disorder. The latest classification, based on proposals from Ketter and Calabrese [37] and Colom and Vieta [38], with the addendum of a fourth subtype for patients with substance abuse, is shown in Table 6.11. Guidelines generally concur in the grading of evidence but disagree on priorities (eg, practically all them point to the value of atypical antipsychotics, lithium, valproate, and carbamazepine in the treatment of mania), but some advise monotherapy and others support combination of two agents. The main reason for these discrepancies has to do with limited evidence from head-to-head trials and the fact that most guidelines seem to pay much more attention to efficacy than to safety and tolerability.

Psychoeducation is also supported by most guidelines as an adjunctive treatment. However, treatment guidelines are rapidly outdated and

Major sources of guideline development

- American Psychiatric Association (APA)
- British Association for Psychopharmacology
- Canadian Network for Mood and Anxiety group
- Danish Psychiatric Association and the Child and Adolescent Psychiatric Association in Denmark
- Department of Veterans Affairs
- European College of Neuropsychopharmacology (ECNP) Consensus Meeting, March 2000, Nice
- Expert Consensus Guideline Series: Medication Treatment of Bipolar Disorder 2000
- National Institute for Health and Clinical Excellence (NICE)
- Texas Medication Algorithm Project
- The Expert Consensus Guidelines for treating depression in bipolar disorder
- The Expert Consensus Panel for Bipolar Disorder
- World Federation of Societies of Biological Psychiatry (WFSBP)

Table 6.10 Major sources of guideline development. Reproduced from Fountoulakis [36].

Classification of mood stabilisers
Class A
• Stabilise 'from **A**bove baseline' • Particularly effective in patients with manic-predominant polarity
Class B
• Stabilise 'from **B**elow baseline' • Particularly effective in patients with depressive-predominant polarity
Class C
• Stabilise 'from the **C**enter' (baseline) • Particularly effective in euthymic patients
Class D
• Stabilise 'from **D**ual morbidity' • Particularly effective in patients with substance abuse

Table 6.11 Classification of mood stabilisers. Based on Kelter and Calabrese [37] and Colom and Vieta [38].

the evidence base tends to relate to registration monotherapy trials that do not accurately reflect routine clinical conditions [36]. The short- and long-term pharmacological management of depressive and manic episodes, including evidence for efficacy, tolerability, and side effects, is reviewed in detail in Chapters 7 and 8.

References

1 Hirschfeld RMA, Bowden CL, Perlis RH, et al. American Psychiatric Association. Practice guideline for the treatment of patients with bipolar disorder [Revision]. *Am J Psychiatry*. 2002;159(suppl 4):1-50.

2 Yatham LN, Kennedy SH, O'Donovan C. Canadian Network for Mood and Anxiety Treatments. Canadian Network for Mood and Anxiety Treatments (CANMAT) guidelines for the management of patients with bipolar disorder: consensus and controversies. *Bipolar Disord*. 2005;7(suppl 3):5-69.

3 Yatham LN, Kennedy SH, O'Donovan C, et al; Guidelines Group, CANMAT. Canadian Network for Mood and Anxiety Treatments (CANMAT) guidelines for the management of patients with bipolar disorder: update 2007. *Bipolar Disord*. 2006;8:721-739.

4 Yatham LN, Kennedy SH, Schaffer A et al. Canadian Network for Mood and Anxiety Treatments (CANMAT) and International Society for Bipolar Disorders (ISBD) collaborative update of CANMAT guidelines for the management of patients with bipolar disorder: update 2009. *Bipolar Disord*. 2009;11:225-255.

5 Goodwin GM; Consensus Group of the British Association for Psychopharmacology. Evidence-based guidelines for treating bipolar disorder: revised second edition—recommendations from the British Association for Psychopharmacology. *J Psychopharmacol*. 2009;23:346-388.

6 National Institute for Health and Excellence (NICE). Bipolar disorder: The management of bipolar disorder in adults, children and adolescents, in primary and secondary care. London: NICE clinical guideline 38. 2006. NICE website. www.nice.org.uk/CG038. Accessed September 18. 2012.

7 Grunze H, Vieta E, Goodwin G, et al. WFSBP Task Force on Treatment Guidelines for Bipolar Disorders. World Federation of Societies of Biological Psychiatry (WFSBP) guidelines for biological treatment of bipolar disorders: update 2010 on the treatment of acute bipolar depression. *World J Biol Psychiatry*. 2010;11:81-109.

8 Grunze H, Vieta E, Goodwin GM, et al. WFSBP Task Force on Treatment Guidelines for Bipolar Disorders. The World Federation of Societies of Biological Psychiatry (WFSBP) guidelines for the biological treatment of bipolar disorders: update 2009 on the treatment of acute mania. *World J Biol Psychiatry*. 2009;10:85-116.

9 Grunze H, Kasper S, Goodwin G, et al. WFSBP Task Force on Treatment Guidelines for Bipolar Disorders. The World Federation of Societies of Biological Psychiatry (WFSBP) guidelines for the biological treatment of bipolar disorders. Part III: maintenance treatment. *World J Biol Psychiatry*. 2004;5:120-135.

10 Sachs G. *Managing Bipolar Affective Disorder*. London, UK: Science Press;2004.

11 Grande I, de Arce R, Jiménez-Arriero MÁ, et al. Patterns of pharmacological maintenance treatment in a community mental health services bipolar disorder cohort study (SIN-DEPRES). *Int J Neuropsychopharmacol*. 2012; epub ahead of print.

12 Vieta E, Günther O, Locklear J, et al. Effectiveness of psychotropic medications in the maintenance phase of bipolar disorder: a meta-analysis of randomized controlled trials. *Int J Neuropsychopharmacol*. 2011;14:1029-1049.

13 Scott J, Colom F, Vieta E. A meta-analysis oaf relapse rates with adjunctive psychological therapies compared to usual psychiatric treatment for bipolar disorder. *Int J Neuropsychopharmacol*. 2007;10:123-129.

14 Miklowitz DJ, Otto MW, Frank E et al. Psychosocial treatments for bipolar depression: a 1-year randomized trial from the Systematic Treatment Enhancement Program. *Arch Gen Psychiatry*. 2007;64:419-426.

15 Colom F, Vieta E, Daban C, et al. Clinical and therapeutic implications of predominant polarity in bipolar disorder. *J Affect Disord*. 2006;93:13-17.

16 Popovic D, Reinares M, Goikoles JM, et al. Polarity index of pharmacological agents used for maintenance treatment of bipolar disorder. *Eur Neuropsychopharmacol*. 2012;22:339-346.

17 Reinares M, Colom F, Sánchez-Moreno J, et al. Impact of caregiver group psychoeducation on the course and outcome of bipolar patients in remission: a randomized controlled trial. *Bipolar Disord*. 2008;10:511-519.

18 Vieta E, Suppes T, Eggens I, et al. Efficacy and safety of quetiapine in combination with lithium or divalproex for maintenance of patients with bipolar I disorder (international trial 126). *J Affect Disord*. 2008;109:251-263.

19 Scott J, Pope M. Self-reported adherence to treatment with mood stabilizers, plasma levels, and psychiatric hospitalization. *Am J Psychiatry*. 2002;159:1927-1929.

20 Colom F, Vieta E, Martinez-Aran A, et al. Clinical factors associated with treatment noncompliance in euthymic bipolar patients. *J Clin Psychiatry*. 2000;61:549-555.

21 Scott J. Predicting medication non-adherence in severe affective disorders. *Acta Neuropsychiatr*. 2000;12:128-130.

22 Muller-Oerlinghausen B, Muser-Causemann B, Volk J. Suicides and parasuicides in a high-risk patient group on and off lithium long-term medication. *J Affect Disord*. 1992;25:261-269.

23 Vieta E. The package of care for patients with bipolar depression. *J Clin Psychiatry*. 2005;66(suppl 5):34-39.

24 Berk M, Berk L, Castle D. A collaborative approach to the treatment alliance in bipolar disorder. *Bipolar Disord*. 2004;6:504-518.

25 Keck PE Jr, McElroy SL, Strakowski SM et al. Compliance with maintenance treatment in bipolar disorder. *Psychopharmacol Bull*. 1997;33:87-91.

26 Colom F, Vieta E. Non-adherence in psychiatric disorders: misbehaviour or clinical feature? *Acta Psychiatr Scand*. 2002;105:161-163.

27 Altshuler L, Suppes T, Black D, et al. Impact of antidepressant discontinuation after acute bipolar depression remission on rates of depressive relapse at 1-year follow-up. *Am J Psychiatry*. 2003;160:1252-1262.

28 Vieta E, Pacchiarotti I, Scott J, et al. Evidence-based research on the efficacy of psychologic interventions in bipolar disorders: a critical review. *Curr Psychiatry Rep*. 2005;7:449-455.

29 Sachs GS, Nierenberg AA, Calabrese JR, et al. Effectiveness of adjunctive antidepressant treatment for bipolar depression. *N Engl J Med*. 2007;356:1711-1722.

30 Baldessarini RJ, Leahy L, Arcona S, et al. Patterns of psychotropic drug prescription for U.S. patients with diagnoses of bipolar disorders. *Psychiatr Serv*. 2007;58:85-91.

31 Vieta E. Role of antidepressants in bipolar depression. *J Clin Psychiatry*. 2010;71:e21.

32 Valentí M, Pacchiarotti I, Rosa AR, et al. Bipolar mixed episodes and antidepressants: a cohort study of bipolar I disorder patients. *Bipolar Disord*. 2011;13:145-154.

33 Goldstein TR, Frye MA, Denicoff KD, et al. Antidepressant discontinuation-related mania: critical prospective observation and theoretical implications in bipolar disorder. *J Clin Psychiatry*. 1999;60:563-567.

34 Miklowitz DJ, Scott J. Psychosocial treatments for bipolar disorder: cost-effectiveness, mediating mechanisms, and future directions. *Bipolar Disord*. 2009;11(suppl 2):110-122.

35 Valentí M, Benabarre A, Bernardo M, et al. Electroconvulsive therapy in the treatment of bipolar depression. *Actas Esp Psiquiatr*. 2007;35:199-207.

36 Fountoulakis KN, Vieta E, Sanchez-Moreno J, et al. Treatment guidelines for bipolar disorder: a critical review. *J Affect Disord*. 2005;86:1-10.

37 Ketter TA, Calabrese JR. Stabilization of mood from below vs above baseline in bipolar disorder: a new nomenclature. *J Clin Psychiatry*. 2002;63:146-151.

38 Colom F, Vieta E. A perspective on the use of psychoeducation, cognitive-behavioral therapy, and interpersonal therapy for bipolar patients. *Bipolar Disord*. 2004;6:480-486.

Chapter 7

Pharmacological management of depressive episodes

Acute depressive episodes

The optimal management of bipolar depression is currently unresolved, although major advances have been recently achieved, and clinical guidelines differ in their recommendations for first- and second-line treatment of acute depressive episodes (Table 7.1) [1–4].

The most commonly advised agents in the acute treatment of bipolar depression are mood stabilisers (eg, lithium), antidepressants (eg, selective serotonin reuptake inhibitors [SSRIs]), and anticonvulsants (eg, lamotrigine, valproate). Newer options, not always reported in guidelines due to the recency of the findings, include atypical antipsychotics (eg, quetiapine, olanzapine). The majority of guidelines advise combination drug therapy for bipolar depression, plus psychotherapy when appropriate.

The choice of which agent to use depends on the patient's age, gender, previous experience with treatment, psychiatric and nonpsychiatric comorbidities, and the potential for abuse. Cost and availability are also factors. It is also important to consider tolerability and utility during the long-term maintenance phase of therapy [5].

Lithium

Lithium is well established from an evidence-based perspective as an effective treatment for acute bipolar depression and has been proven superior to placebo, with response rates of up to 80% in nine methodically limited randomized controlled trials [6]. Despite the results of those old

E. Vieta, *Managing Bipolar Disorder in Clinical Practice*, DOI: 10.1007/978-1-908517-94-4_7, © Springer Healthcare 2013

Comparison of guideline recommendations for the treatment of acute bipolar depression

	First line	Second line	Not recommended
American Psychiatric Association, 2002 [1]	Lithium *or* lamotrigine *or* lithium + antidepressant ECT	Combination of first-line agents ECT	
Canadian Network for Mood and Anxiety Disorders (CANMAT) and International Society for Bipolar Disorders (ISBD), 2009 [2]	Lithium, lamotrigine, quetiapine, quetiapine XR, lithium or valproate + SSRI or bupropion, lithium + valproate, olanzapine + SSRI	Quetiapine + SSRI, valproate, lithium or valproate + lamotrigine, adjunctive monotherapy Psychotherapy ECT	Gabapentin, aripiprazole
British Association for Psychopharmacology, 2009 [3]	*Severe:* Quetiapine, lamotrigine, possibly an antipsychotic ECT *Milder:* Quetiapine, lamotrigine	SSRI + antimanic (lithium, valproate, antipsychotic) Psychotherapy ECT	
World Federation of Societies of Biological Psychiatry, 2010 [4]	Quetiapine, fluoxetine, lamotrigine, olanzapine, valproate, olanzapine + fluoxetine, lamotrigine + lithium	Augmentation strategies Psychotherapy ECT	Paroxetine, aripiprazole, ziprasidone

Table 7.1 Comparison of guideline recommendations for the treatment of acute bipolar depression. ECT, electroconvulsive therapy; SSRI, selective serotonin reuptake inhibitor.

trials, however, its efficacy, specifically against acute bipolar depression, has been questioned [7] and in a recent trial it did not separate from placebo, even though quetiapine did [8]. Nevertheless, it remains a potential comparator for new studies in bipolar disorder. The disadvantages of lithium in the acute treatment of bipolar depression are its slow onset of action (usually between 1 and 2 months) and the side-effect profile, which includes weight gain, tremor, gastrointestinal disturbances, and lethargy.

Lithium has also been evaluated in combination with antidepressants. A study of outpatients with bipolar depression compared the efficacy of lithium monotherapy with combined lithium and paroxetine and combined lithium and imipramine. Overall, the combination therapies were not superior to lithium monotherapy. However, at lithium blood levels below 0.8 mmol/L, both the paroxetine and imipramine combinations were superior to lithium alone [9]. Antidepressants may thus be useful adjunctive therapy for patients who cannot tolerate high serum levels of lithium.

Lithium may also be used with an anticonvulsant. In a small, randomized controlled trial, the combination of lithium plus valproate was as effective as lithium or valproate plus paroxetine in improving depressive symptoms [10]. Paroxetine was significantly better tolerated than the combination of two mood stabilisers, suggesting that adding paroxetine to a mood stabiliser might have more clinical utility than adding a second mood stabiliser, but paroxetine has failed to separate from placebo in several trials in bipolar depression, including a monotherapy one [11]. The combination of lithium and lamotrigine proved effective for bipolar depression in a placebo-controlled trial [12]. This combination would have the advantage of providing longer-term protection according to the results of a long-term monotherapy study, in which lithium was better than placebo in the prevention of mania, and lamotrigine was better than placebo in the prevention of depression [13].

Antidepressants

There is general agreement that antidepressant monotherapy should be avoided in view of the potential for mood switching and cycle acceleration. The coadministration of a traditional mood-stabilizing agent does not completely eliminate these risks, however, and the optimal use of antidepressants continues to be debated [14–17]. In a recent large effectiveness trial conducted within the Systematic Treatment Enhancement Program for Bipolar Disorder (STEP-BD) program, adjunctive antidepressants were not better than placebo, although there was no signal of switch [17]. Table 7.2 summarizes the side effects, dosing, advantages, and disadvantages of antidepressants commonly used for bipolar disorder [18].

A meta-analysis of antidepressants for bipolar depression found that active therapy was superior to placebo with respect to clinical response and remission [19]. The analysis included 12 trials and 1088 randomized

Comparison of antidepressants commonly used for bipolar disorder

Drug	Sed	AC	HT	SD	Advantages
Imipramine	+++	+++	++	++	
Desipramine	–/++	++	+	+	Can be activating
Amitriptyline	++++	++++	+++	+++	
Nortriptyline	++	++	+	++	Mildly sedating, least hypotension of TCAs
Doxepin	++++	+++	++	+++	Sedating, effective antihistamine; effective H_2-receptor blocker
Protriptyline	–/+	+++	++	+	Useful for sleep apnea, most activation of TCAs
Fluoxetine	–/+	–	–	+++	Few need >20 mg, activating, very safe in overdose, few experience weight gain
Sertraline	–/+	–	–	+++	Fewer drug–drug interactions, activating, very safe in overdose, few experience weight gain
Paroxetine	–/++	?/++	–	+++	Short half-life, no metabolites, jitters less likely, may be less mania
Bupropion	–/+	–	–	–	Activating, few experience weight gain, less therapy-emergent mania, no sexual dysfunction
Escitalopram	–/+	–	–	+	Few drug–drug interactions, activating, very safe in overdose, few experience weight gain

Table 7.2 Comparison of antidepressants commonly used for bipolar disorder.
AC, anticholinergic; bid, twice daily; H2, histamine 2; HT, hypotension; IR, immediate release; qam, every morning; qhs, every night at bedtime; SD, sexual dysfunction; sed, sedation; SR, sustained release; TCA, tricyclic anti-depressant; tid, three times daily; UED, usual effective dose; USD, usual starting dose; XL, extended release; –, none/infrequent; +, common; ++, frequent; +++, most frequent; ?, questionable/possible. Reproduced from Sachs [18].

patients on short-term treatment with a range of antidepressants, including fluoxetine, paroxetine, imipramine, tranylcypromine, deprenyl, desipramine, and bupropion. Overall, antidepressants did not induce more switching to mania than placebo. However, the risk of switching was significantly higher with tricyclic agents than with SSRIs or monoamine oxidase inhibitors (MAOIs) (10% versus 3.2%), leading the authors to recommend avoiding tricyclics as first-line agents in bipolar depression.

Venlafaxine was compared with paroxetine in a 6-week randomized trial in patients with breakthrough depression despite treatment with a mood stabiliser [20]. Both treatments significantly improved depressive symptomatology with no difference in tolerability. However, the switch rate to hypomania or mania was higher with venlafaxine than with paroxetine (13% versus 3%). These results have been confirmed in a randomized trial comparing bupropion, sertraline, and venlafaxine as

Disadvantages	USD (mg)	UED (mg)
Seizure risk 0.1%	25–50 qhs–bid	150–300
Activation may be excessive, jitters, insomnia	25–50 qam/qhs/bid	150–300
Sedation, weight gain, hypotension	25–50 qhs–bid	150–300
Seizure risk 0.1%	10–25 qhs–bid	75–150
Most weight gain	25–50 qhs–bid	150–300
Jitters, insomnia, longest half-life TCA	5–10 qam–bid	15–60
Headache, nausea, rash, jitters, seizure risk 0.2%	10–20 qam	10–60
Headache, nausea, rash, jitters	50 qam	50–200
Sedation, anticholinergic like, drug–drug interactions	20 qam or qhs	20–50
Seizure risk 0.1% Confusional state	IR 75–100 qam/bid; SR/XL 100–150 qam	IR 100 tid 150 bid/tid; SR 150–200 bid; XL 300–450 qam
Nausea, insomnia	10	10–20 qam

adjuncts to mood stabilisers [21]. The only adequately powered, placebo-controlled trial of an SSRI as monotherapy in bipolar depression did not demonstrate neither efficacy or switch risk, although the dose was low (paroxetine 20 mg/day) [11]. Newer antidepressants, such as agomelatine, are being actively researched in this indication [22].

Anticonvulsants

Lamotrigine has demonstrated efficacy in treating bipolar depression in two out of four randomized placebo-controlled trials [12,23,24], suggesting that its real strength lies in long-term treatment. A recent meta-analysis as well as an analysis of five other randomized, placebo-controlled trials confirmed these findings, showing a modest clinical benefit with lamotrigine therapy [25,26]. Lamotrigine was not associated with an increased risk of switching to mania. It has a slow onset of action of around 3 weeks and is generally well tolerated, although slow dose escalation is necessary to avoid the risk of allergic reactions, including severe rash.

There is some evidence supporting the use of valproate in acute bipolar depression. Two small placebo-controlled trials found that valproate mono-therapy was well tolerated and superior to placebo in bipolar depressed patients [27,28]. Moreover, valproate has antimanic properties and there-fore may protect against mania when treating depression, which is an advantage over antidepressants and over lamotrigine, and is generally better tolerated than antipsychotics [29,30]. However, larger trials will need to be conducted to fully determine valproate's effectiveness [25].

Carbamazepine has been poorly studied in the treatment of acute bipolar depression. One placebo-controlled study in patients with bipolar disorder suggested moderate efficacy [31], but others did not replicate this [32,33]. Carbamazepine cannot therefore be recommended as mono-therapy for bipolar depression [25]. It can also increase the metabolism of several antidepressants and atypical antipsychotics, which can make monitoring treatment difficult. Acute levetiracetam adjunctive mono-therapy has been studied in one clinical trials, but it was not superior to placebo [25,34].

Atypical antipsychotics

Evidence is rapidly accumulating in support of some atypical antipsy-chotics in the treatment of acute bipolar depression [35,36]. An 8-week placebo-controlled study in patients with bipolar I disorder found that olanzapine alone or in combination with fluoxetine was significantly more effective than placebo and did not cause switching into mania or hypomania [37]. The response was greatest in the combination therapy group, with a 48.8% remission rate, and the combination of olanzapine plus fluoxetine was subsequently licensed in the US for the acute treat-ment of bipolar depression. In this study, side effects included somnolence, weight gain, increased appetite, dry mouth, asthenia, and diarrhea [37].

Quetiapine monotherapy has also shown efficacy for the treat-ment of bipolar I or II depression. In a large, randomized, double-blind, placebo-controlled trial, quetiapine significantly improved nine of ten core features of depression and was generally well tolerated at doses of 300 and 600 mg/day [38]. Improvements were seen within 1 week and were maintained throughout the study. Moreover, the incidence of treatment-emergent mania was not increased versus placebo. Side effects were dose-related and included dry mouth, sedation, somnolence, dizziness, and constipation [38]. These positive results were subsequently confirmed in a similar trial [39] and across bipolar subtypes, such as bipolar II disorder [40] and rapid cyclers [41]. Two more recent trials replicated the same findings and had lithium [8] and paroxetine [11] as active comparators. Neither lithium nor paroxetine was able to beat placebo, although quetiapine did. Two other trials found that quetiapine extended release was also superior to placebo in bipolar depression [39,42]. These findings were sufficient for the World Federation of Societies of Biological Psychiatry to rate quetiapine as its top treatment choice for acute bipolar depression [4,43].

The data have not been so positive with other antipsychotics, however: risperidone was not efficacious in an STEP-BD comparative trial with inositol and lamotrigine [44], and two placebo-controlled trials of ari-piprazole monotherapy failed, although there was a significant separation from placebo from week 1 to week 6, which was lost at weeks 7 and 8 [45]. Attending to these data, we have hypothesized a model for the mechanism of action of atypical antipsychotics that might explain the treatment response pattern and its timing (Figure 7.1).

Long-term maintenance therapy

The goals of treatment in bipolar depression are to resolve depressive symptoms and establish a stable mood. In general, what makes patients well is likely to keep them well too, but there are very few long-term trials in bipolar disorder with bipolar depression as the index episode and, for some compounds, such as antidepressants, it is very unclear if long-term treatment is either good or bad. In fact, most guidelines recommend that antidepressants should be discontinued within 3–6 months of remission [46,47]. The rationale for this approach is influenced by a concern that continued antidepressant treatment might induce switches into mania or cycle acceleration. Thus, in contrast to the long-term use

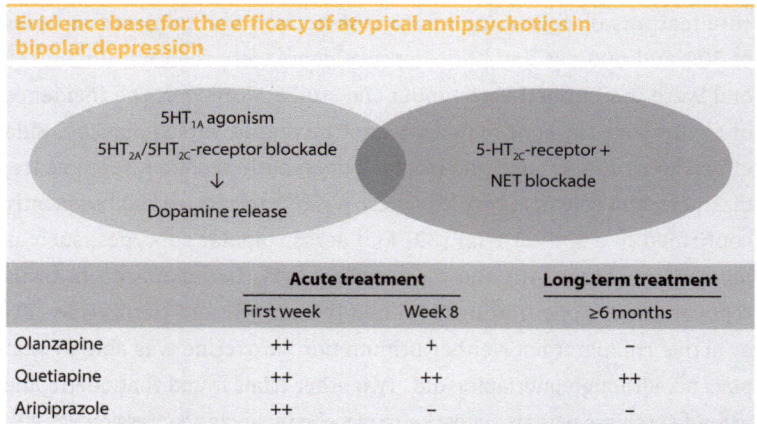

Figure 7.1 Evidence base for the efficacy of atypical antipsychotics in bipolar depression.
Potential mechanisms of action involved in immediate versus mid- and long-term antidepressant
efficacy of atypical antipsychotics in bipolar depression. 5-HT, 5-hydroxytryptamine receptor 2C;
NET, norepinephrine transporter. ++, at least one good placebo-controlled trial showing clinically
significant effects; +, at least one placebo-controlled trial showing some effect; –, evidence of
a lack of clinically significant effects.

of mood stabilisers, antidepressant treatment is generally advised on a
temporary basis only [48].

In this scenario, the duration of antidepressant treatment is determined by past history in terms of liability for mood destabilization, and
the ability of the patient to tolerate gradual antidepressant discontinuation
without a return of symptoms. However, a non-randomized study suggested that stopping the antidepressant too early after a response might
be associated with a higher risk of relapse [49], and patients should be
monitored closely for re-emergence of depressive symptoms as well as
mania induced by antidepressant discontinuation [50].

As a response to the relative paucity of long-term trials, a meta-
analysis was conducted to compare the effectiveness of long-term maintenance agents through the number needed to treat (NNT) measurement.
Lamotrigine, lithium, and quetiapine alone and lithium + valproate had
single-digit NNTs and were thus determined to be effective in preventing
depressive relapses [51].

There is some, albeit limited, evidence to suggest that long-term
maintenance therapy may be helpful after an acute bipolar depressive

episode. A retrospective chart review found that lithium reduced depressive morbidity in patients with bipolar I and II disorders, and that starting lithium maintenance earlier predicted greater improvement [52]. Lithium is also thought to have specific antisuicidal properties [53,54]. However, several meta-analyses have suggested that lithium is only marginally effective in preventing depressive relapses [55–58].

Practical issues relating to long-term lithium use include dosing, tolerability, and withdrawal. Relapse rates are lower in patients with plasma levels maintained at 0.8–1.0 mmol/L than in those at 0.4–0.6 mmol/L [57], and daily dosing is more effective than dosing every other day [59]. However, side effects may prevent the long-term use of high lithium doses [60]. In addition, sudden discontinuation of lithium may provoke a relapse [61,62], and reinstituting lithium may not always be effective [63]. Lithium should thus always be tapered slowly over weeks or even months. Some patients may also develop treatment resistance after previously having a good response to treatment [63].

Anticonvulsants may be considered as maintenance treatment following bipolar depression in view of their mood-stabilizing properties. In an 18-month, randomized, double-blind study in patients with bipolar I disorder who had recently suffered a depressive episode, lamotrigine and lithium were both superior to placebo in preventing any mood episode. Lamotrigine, but not lithium, was superior to placebo in preventing a depressive episode, while lithium, but not lamotrigine, was superior to placebo in preventing a manic, hypomanic, or mixed episode [13]. In another study, the combination of lamotrigine and lithium had superior efficacy versus placebo over the long term, for up to 68 weeks [64].

Valproate has also shown potential for preventing recurrent depressive episodes. A 12-month, randomized, placebo-controlled study in outpatients with bipolar I disorder found that valproate, but not lithium, was superior to placebo in preventing depressive relapses [65]. However, this was a secondary analysis and neither valproate nor lithium was superior to placebo with respect to the study's primary endpoint (time to recurrence of any mood episode).

Olanzapine in combination with fluoxetine (OFC) was compared with lamotrigine in a 6-month randomized trial [37]. Both strategies were similarly effective in the long term but OFC had a much faster onset of action; tolerability, however, was overall better for lamotrigine. Olanzapine was also studied as monotherapy in patients with bipolar I disorder who had previously responded to acute olanzapine treatment. Time to relapse was significantly longer in patients given the active agent than in patients given placebo, with fewer instances of symptomatic relapse [66].

Quetiapine is currently the best studied compound in this indication, with two positive, adjunctive, long-term studies showing effective prevention of both mania and depression in patients with an index depressive episode (the trials were also positive for patients with manic and mixed index episode), and two monotherapy 1-year studies as continuation of the short-term ones called EMBOLDEN I and II [8,11], showing effective prevention of depressive recurrences. A third monotherapy study found that treatment with either quetiapine or lithium alone increased time to recurrence of depressive events, compared with placebo [67].

Table 7.3 compares the first- and second-line recommendations for maintenance therapy in various clinical guidelines [1–3,68]. Once all of

Comparison of guideline recommendations for maintenance treatment of bipolar depression		
	First line	**Second line**
American Psychiatric Association, 2002 [1]	Lithium *or* valproate Possibly carbamazepine, lamotrigine *or* oxcarbazepine Continue the treatment	Combination of first-line agents ECT Antipsychotics should be discontinued
World Federation of Societies of Biological Psychiatry, 2004 [68]	Lamotrigine, antidepressant + mood stabiliser Possibly valproate *or* carbamazepine	Risperidone (add-on) Psychotherapy ECT
Canadian Network for Mood and Anxiety Disorders (CANMAT) and International Society for Bipolar Disorders (ISBD), 2009 [2]	Lithium, lamotrigine, valproate, olanzapine, quetiapine, lithium or valproate + quetiapine, adjunctive risperidone, adjunctive ziprasidone	Risperidone (add-on), carbamazepine, combination of first-line agents Psychotherapy
British Association for Psychopharmacology, 2009 [3]	Lithium, quetiapine, lamotrigine	Lithium, combination therapy Psychotherapy

Table 7.3 Comparison of guideline recommendations for maintenance treatment of bipolar depression. ECT, electroconvulsive therapy.

these guidelines are updated, there may be critical changes due to the inclusion of the quetiapine data.

References

1   Fountoulakis KN, Vieta E, Sanchez-Moreno J, et al. Treatment guidelines for bipolar disorder: a critical review. *J Affect Disord*. 2005;86:1-10.

2   Yatham LN, Kennedy SH, Schaffer A, et al. Canadian Network for Mood and Anxiety Treatments (CANMAT) and International Society for Bipolar Disorders (ISBD) collaborative update of CANMAT guidelines for the management of patients with bipolar disorder: update 2009. *Bipolar Disord*. 2009;11:225-255.

3   Goodwin GM; Consensus Group of the British Association for Psychopharmacology. Evidence-based guidelines for treating bipolar disorder: revised second edition — recommendations from the British Association for Psychopharmacology. *J Psychopharmacol*. 2009;23:346-388.

4   Grunze H, Vieta E, Goodwin G, et al. WFSBP Task Force on Treatment Guidelines for Bipolar Disorders. World Federation of Societies of Biological Psychiatry (WFSBP) guidelines for biological treatment of bipolar disorders: update 2010 on the treatment of acute bipolar depression. *World J Biol Psychiatry*. 2010;11:81-109.

5   Bauer M, Ritter P, Grunze H, et al. Treatment options for acute depression in bipolar disorder. *Bipolar Disord*. 2012;14(suppl 2):37-50.

6   Zornberg GL, Pope HG Jr. Treatment of depression in bipolar disorder: new directions for research. *J Clin Psychopharmacol*. 1993;13:397-408.

7   Bhagwagar Z, Goodwin GM, McElroy SL, Bauer M *et al*, EMBOLDEN I (Trial 001) Investigators. The role of lithium in the treatment of bipolar depression. *Clin Neurosci Res*. 2002;2:222-227.

8   Young AH, McElroy SL, Bauer M et al; EMBOLDEN I (Trial 001) Investigators. A double-blind, placebo-controlled study of quetiapine and lithium monotherapy in adults in the acute phase of bipolar depression (EMBOLDEN I). *J Clin Psychiatry*. 2010;71:150-162.

9   Nemeroff CB, Evans DL, Gyulai L, et al. Double-blind, placebo-controlled comparison of imipramine and paroxetine in the treatment of bipolar depression. *Am J Psychiatry*. 2001;158:906-912.

10 Young L, Joffe R, Robb J, et al. Double-blind comparison of addition of a second mood stabilizer versus an antidepressant to an initial mood stabilizer for treatment of patients with bipolar depression. *Am J Psychiatry*. 2000;157:124-126.

11 McElroy S, SL, Weisler RH, Chang W, et al; EMBOLDEN II (Trial D1447C00134) Investigators. A double-blind, placebo-controlled study of quetiapine and paroxetine in adults with bipolar depression (EMBOLDEN II). *J Clin Psychiatry*. 2010;71:163-174.

12 van der Loos ML, Mulder PGH, Hartong EG ThM, et al; the LamLit Study Group. Efficacy and safety of lamotrigine as add-on to lithium in the treatment of bipolar depression: a multicenter, double-blind, placebo-controlled trial. *J Clin Psychiatry*. 2009;70:223-231.

13 Calabrese JR, Bowden CL, Sachs G, et al. A placebo-controlled 18-month trial of lamotrigine and lithium maintenance treatment in recently depressed patients with bipolar I disorder. *J Clin Psychiatry*. 2003;64:1013-1024.

14 Ghaemi SN, Hsu DJ, Soldani F, et al. Antidepressants in bipolar disorder: the case for caution. *Bipolar Disord*. 2003;5:421-433.

15 Vieta E. Case for caution, case for action. *Bipolar Disord*. 2003;5:434-435.

16 Goldberg JF, Truman CJ. Antidepressant-induced mania: an overview of current controversies. *Bipolar Disord*. 2003;5:407-420.

17 Vieta E. Overcoming the current approach in bipolar disorder research: towards DSM-V and beyond. *J Psychopharmacol*. 2008;22:406-407.

18 Sachs G. *Managing Bipolar Affective Disorder*. London, UK: Science Press; 2004.

19 Gijsman HJ, Geddes JR, Rendell JM et al. Antidepressants for bipolar depression: a systematic review of randomized, controlled trials. *Am J Psychiatry*. 2004;161:1537-1547.

20 Vieta E, Martinez-Aran A, Goikolea JM, et al. A randomized trial comparing paroxetine and venlafaxine in the treatment of bipolar depressed patients taking mood stabilizers. *J Clin Psychiatry*. 2002;63:508-512.

21 Leverich GS, Altshuler LL, Frye MA, et al. Risk of switch in mood polarity to hypomania or mania in patients with bipolar depression during acute and continuation trials of venlafaxine, sertraline, and bupropion as adjuncts to mood stabilizers. *Am J Psychiatry*. 2006;163:232-239.

22 Calabrese JR, Guelfi JD, Perdrizet-Chevallier C, Agomelatine Bipolar Study Group. Agomelatine adjunctive therapy for acute bipolar depression: preliminary open data. *Bipolar Disord*. 2007; 9:628–635.

23 Calabrese J, Bowden C, Sachs G, et al. A double-blind placebo-controlled study of lamotrigine monotherapy in outpatients with bipolar I depression. Lamictal 602 Study Group. *J Clin Psychiatry*. 1999;60:79-88.

24 Calabrese JR, Huffman RF, White RL, et al. Lamotrigine in the acute treatment of bipolar depression: results of five double-blind, placebo-controlled clinical trials. *Bipolar Disord*. 2008;10:323-333.

25 Reinares M, Rosa AR, Franco C et al. A systematic review on the role of anticonvulsants in the treatment of acute bipolar depression. *Int J Neuropsychopharmacol*. 2012; [epub ahead of print].

26 Geddes JR, Calabrese JR, Goodwin GM. Lamotrigine for treatment of bipolar depression: independent meta-analysis and meta-regression of individual patient data from five randomised trials. *Br J Psychiatry*. 2009;194:4-9.

27 Davis LL, Bartolucci A, Petty F. Divalproex in the treatment of bipolar depression: a placebo-controlled study. *J Affect Disord*. 2005;85:259-266.

28 Ghaemi SN, Gilmer WS, Goldberg JF, et al. Divalproex in the treatment of acute bipolar depression: a preliminary double-blind, randomized, placebo-controlled pilot study. *J Clin Psychiatry*. 2007;68:1840-1844.

29 Tohen M, Vieta E, Goodwin GM et al. Olanzapine versus divalproex versus placebo in the treatment of mild to moderate mania: a randomized, 12-week, double-blind study. *J Clin Psychiatry*. 2008;69:1776-1789.

30 Torrent C, Amann B, Sánchez-Moreno J et al. Weight gain in bipolar disorder: pharmacological treatment as a contributing factor. *Acta Psychiatr Scand*. 2008;118:4-18.

31 Ballenger JC. The clinical use of carbamazepine in affective disorder. *J Clin Psychiat*. 1988;49(suppl 4):13-19.

32 Small JG. Anticonvulsants in affective disorders. *Psychopharmacol Bull*. 1990;26:25-36.

33 Zhang Z-J, Kang W-H, Tan Q-R, et al. Adjunctive herbal medicine with carbamazepine for bipolar disorders: a double-blind, randomized, placebo-controlled study. *J Psychiatry Res*. 2007;41:360-369.

34 Saricicek A, Maloney K, Muralidharan A, et al. Levetiracetam in the management of bipolar depression: a randomized, double-blind, placebo-controlled trial. *J Clin Psychiatry*. 2011;72:744-750.

35 Vieta E. Atypical antipsychotics in the treatment of mood disorders. *Curr Opin Psychiatry*. 2003;16:23-27.

36 Yatham LN, Goldstein JM, Vieta E, et al. Atypical antipsychotics in bipolar depression: potential mechanisms of action. *J Clin Psychiatry*. 2005;66(suppl 5):40-48.

37 Tohen M, Vieta E, Calabrese J, et al. Efficacy of olanzapine and olanzapine–fluoxetine combination in the treatment of bipolar I depression. *Arch Gen Psychiatry*. 2003;60:1079-1088.

38 Calabrese JR, Keck PE Jr, Macfadden W, et al. A randomized, double-blind, placebo-controlled trial of quetiapine in the treatment of bipolar I or II depression. *Am J Psychiatry*. 2005;162:1351-1360.

39 Thase ME, Macfadden W, Weisler RH, et al; BOLDER II Study Group. Efficacy of quetiapine monotherapy in bipolar I and II depression: a double-blind, placebo-controlled study (the BOLDER II study). *J Clin Psychopharmacol*. 2006;26:600-609.

40 Suppes T, Hirschfeld RM, Vieta E et al. Quetiapine for the treatment of bipolar II depression: Analysis of data from two randomized, double-blind, placebo-controlled studies. *World J Biol Psychiatry*. 2007;11:1-14.

41 Vieta E, Calabrese JR, Goikolea JM, et al, BOLDER Study Group. Quetiapine monotherapy in the treatment of patients with bipolar I or II depression and a rapid-cycling disease course: a randomized, double-blind, placebo-controlled study. *Bipolar Disord*. 2007;9:413-425.

42 Suppes T, Datto C, Minkwitz M, et al. Effectiveness of the extended release formulations of quetiapine as monotherapy for the treatment of acute bipolar depression. *J Affect Disord*. 2010;121:106-115.

43 Vieta E, Grunze H. Bipolar disorder—a focus on depression. *N Engl J Med*. 2011;364:1581.

44 Nierenberg AA, Ostacher MJ, Calabrese JR, et al. Treatment-resistant bipolar depression: a STEP-BD equipoise randomized effectiveness trial of antidepressant augmentation with lamotrigine, inositol, or risperidone. *Am J Psychiatry*. 2006;163:210-216.

45 Thase ME, Jonas A, Khan A et al. Aripiprazole monotherapy in nonpsychotic bipolar I depression: results of 2 randomized, placebo-controlled studies. *J Clin Psychopharmacol*. 2008;28:13-20.

46 Frances A, Kahn D, Carpenter S, et al. The expert consensus guidelines for treating depression in bipolar disorder. *J Clin Psychiatry*. 1998;59(suppl 4):S73-S79.

47 Yatham L, Kusumakar V, Parikh S, et al. Bipolar depression: treatment options. *Can J Psychiatry*. 1997;42(suppl 2):S87-S91.

48 Montgomery SA, Schatzberg AF, Guelfi JD, et al. Pharmacotherapy of depression and mixed states in bipolar disorder. *J Affect Disord*. 2000;59(suppl 1):S39-S56.

49 Altshuler L, Suppes T, Black D, et al. Impact of antidepressant discontinuation after acute bipolar depression remission on rates of depressive relapse at 1-year follow-up. *Am J Psychiatry*. 2003;160:1252-1262.

50 Goldstein TR, Frye MA, Denicoff KD et al. Antidepressant discontinuation-related mania: critical prospective observation and theoretical implications in bipolar disorder. *J Clin Psychiatry*. 1999;60:563-567.

51 Popovic D, Reinares M, Amann B, et al. Number needed to treat analyses of drugs used for maintenance treatment of bipolar disorder. *Psychopharmacology (Berl)*. 2011;213:657-667.

52 Tondo L, Baldessarini RJ, Hennen J, et al. Lithium maintenance treatment of depression and mania in bipolar I and bipolar II disorders. *Am J Psychiatry*. 1998;155:638-645.

53 Ahrens B, Muller-Oerlinghausen B. Does lithium exert an independent antisuicidal effect? *Pharmacopsychiatry*. 2001;34:132-136.

54 Goodwin FK, Fireman B, Simon GE, et al. Suicide risk in bipolar disorder during treatment with lithium and divalproex. *JAMA*. 2003;290:1467-1473.

55 Burgess S, Geddes J, Hawton K, et al. Lithium for maintenance treatment of mood disorders. *Cochrane Database Syst Rev*. 2001;(3)CD003013.

56 Davis JM, Janicak PG, Hogan DM. Mood stabilizers in the prevention of recurrent affective disorders: a metaanalysis. *Acta Psychiatr Scand*. 1999;100:406-417.

57 Geddes J, Burgess S, Hawton K, et al. Long-term lithium therapy for bipolar disorder: systematic review and meta-analysis of randomized controlled trials. *Am J Psychiatry*. 2004;161:217-222.

58 Nivoli AMA, Murru A, Vieta E. Lithium: still a cornerstone in the long-term treatment of bipolar disorder? *Neuropsychobiology*. 2010;62:27-35.

59 Jensen HV, Plenge P, Mellerup ET et al. Lithium prophylaxis of manic-depressive disorder: daily lithium dosing schedule versus every second day. *Acta Psychiatr Scand*. 1995;92:69-74.

60 Fountoulakis KN, Vieta E, Bouras C, et al. A systematic review of existing data on long-term lithium therapy: neuroprotective or neurotoxic? *Int J Neuropsychopharmacol*. 2008;11:269-287.

61 Mander AJ, Loudon JB. Rapid recurrence of mania following abrupt discontinuation of lithium. *Lancet.* 1988;2:15-17.

62 Goodwin GM. Recurrence of mania after lithium withdrawal. Implications for the use of lithium in the treatment of bipolar affective disorder. *Br J Psychiatry.* 1994;164:149-152.

63 Post RM. Acquired lithium resistance revisited: discontinuation-induced refractoriness versus tolerance. *J Affect Disord.* 2012;140:6-13.

64 van der Loos MLM, Mulder P, Hartong EG ThM, et al. Long-term outcome of bipolar depressed patients receiving lamotrigine as add-on to lithium with the possibility of the addition of paroxetine in nonresponders: a randomized, placebo-controlled trial with a novel design. *Bipolar Disord.* 2011;13:111-117.

65 Bowden CL, Calabrese JR, McElroy SL, et al. A randomized, placebo-controlled 12-month trial of divalproex and lithium in treatment of outpatients with bipolar I disorder. Divalproex Maintenance Study Group. *Arch Gen Psychiatry.* 2000;57:481-489.

66 Tohen M, Calabrese JR, Sachs GS, et al. Randomized, placebo-controlled trial of olanzapine as maintenance therapy in patients with bipolar I disorder responding to acute treatment with olanzapine. *Am J Psychiatry.* 2006;163:247-256.

67 Weisler RH, Nolen WA, Neijber A et al; Trial 144 Study Investigators. Continuation of quetiapine versus switching to placebo or lithium for maintenance treatment of bipolar I disorder (Trial 144: a randomized controlled study). *J Clin Psychiatry.* 2011;72:1452-1464.

68 Grunze H, Kasper S, Goodwin G, et al; WFSBP Task Force on Treatment Guidelines for Bipolar Disorders. The World Federation of Societies of Biological Psychiatry (WFSBP) guidelines for the biological treatment of bipolar disorders. Part III: maintenance treatment. *World J Biol Psychiatry.* 2004;5:120-135.

Chapter 8

Pharmacological management of manic episodes

Acute manic, hypomanic, and mixed episodes

The goals of treatment of an acute manic or mixed episode are to alleviate symptoms and allow a return to usual levels of psychosocial functioning. Achieving rapid control of agitation, aggression, poor judgement, and impulsivity is particularly important to ensure the safety of patients and those around them and to allow the establishment of a therapeutic alliance.

Although diagnostic criteria allow bipolar mood episodes to be defined as hypomanic, manic, or mixed, it can be difficult to reliably discriminate between them. The degree of mood elevation itself is not the decisive factor in choosing among the three diagnoses; instead, the degree of impairment and behavioral disturbance, as evidenced by aggression, agitation, psychosis, poor judgment, and social or occupational dysfunction, is the usual precipitant of clinical attention and hence the primary target of intervention. In practical terms, therefore, bipolar I disorder patients presenting with a hypomanic, manic, or mixed episode can usually be managed with a common 'acute mood elevation' strategy.

The most widely used medications in the acute setting are lithium, some anticonvulsants (valproate, carbamazepine), standard antipsychotics (eg, haloperidol, chlorpromazine), atypical antipsychotics (eg, quetiapine, olanzapine, risperidone, ziprasidone, aripiprazole, amisulpride, clozapine), and benzodiazepines (eg, lorazepam, clonazepam).

The choice of initial treatment is influenced by the patient's current and prior medication history, the need for rapid resolution of agitation

E. Vieta, *Managing Bipolar Disorder in Clinical Practice*,
DOI: 10.1007/978-1-908517-94-4_8, © Springer Healthcare 2013

and aggression, the characteristics of the manic episode, and the presence of rapid cycling, as well as the patient's own willingness to accept particular therapies and routes of administration. Whenever possible, oral therapy should be offered first, but intramuscular injections are an alternative if oral therapy cannot be reliably administered. Clinical features that can help guide initial treatment choices are summarized in Table 8.1 [1].

Clinical guidelines show some differences in their recommendations for the first- and second-line treatment of acute mania, as summarized in Table 8.2 [2–5]. The strength of evidence supporting the various options, as monotherapy and in combination, is given in Tables 8.3 and 8.4 [1,3],

Clinical factors that predict treatment response		
Agent	**Predictors of response**	**Predictors of non-response**
Lithium	Elated mania	Mixed state
	Previous response to lithium	Rapid cycling
	Mania–depression–euthymia course	Depression–mania–euthymia course
	No neurological impairment	Presence of depressive symptoms
	No psychotic symptoms	Multiple episodes
	No substance abuse	No family history
	Few episodes of illness	
Valproate	Rapid cycling	Comorbid personality disorders
	Mixed state	More severe mania
	Multiple prior mood episodes	
	Irritable-dysphonic subtype	
	Secondary mania	
	Comorbid substance abuse	
Carbamazepine	Mixed state	Rapid cycling
	Increased severity of acute mania	>10-year history of illness
	No family history of mood disorders	
	Early age of onset	
	Course dominated by manic episodes	
Atypical antipsychotics	Early age of onset	
	No prior substance abuse	
	No prior antipsychotic treatment	
	Rapid cycling	

Table 8.1 Clinical factors that predict treatment response. Reproduced with permission from Yatham et al [1].

and specific approaches are discussed below, but it must be kept in mind that some of these guidelines are out of date.

Lithium

Lithium has been used in the treatment of acute bipolar mania for over 50 years, and has demonstrated superiority over placebo in several controlled clinical trials [6]. In these studies, the percentage of patients showing at least moderate improvement after 2–3 weeks of treatment ranged from 40% to 80%. Lithium appears to be most effective in patients with classic (euphoric) mania, while response rates are relatively poor in mixed states or rapid cycling [7].

Comparison of guideline recommendations for the treatment of acute bipolar mania			
	First line	**Second line**	**Not recommended**
American Psychiatric Association, 2002 [2]	*Severe:* lithium or valproate + antipsychotic *Mild-moderate:* lithium, valproate, olanzapine	Various combinations of two first-line agents ECT	
Canadian Network for Mood and Anxiety Disorders (CANMAT) and International Society for Bipolar Disorders (ISBD), 2009 [3]	Lithium, valproate, olanzapine, risperidone, quetiapine, quetiapine XR, aripiprazole, ziprasidone, lithium or valproate + antipsychotic	Carbamazepine, asenapine, paliperidone, lithium + valproate, lithium or valproate + asenapine Psychotherapy ECT	Monotherapy with gabapentin, topiramate, lamotrigine, verapamil, tiagabine Risperidone or olanzapine + carbamazepine
British Association for Psychopharmacology, 2009 [4]	*Severe:* Antipsychotic, valproate, possibly IM benzodiazepine ECT *Milder:* Antipsychotic, valproate, lithium, carbamazepine	Taper and discontinue antidepressants Consider clozapine Psychotherapy ECT	
World Federation of Societies of Biological Psychiatry, 2009 [5]	Lithium, carbamazepine, valproate, aripiprazole, olanzapine, quetiapine, risperidone, asenapine	Ziprasidone, haloperidol, combinations of first-line agents ECT	Gabapentin, topiramate, lamotrigine, tiagabine, pregabalin

Table 8.2 Comparison of guideline recommendations for the treatment of acute bipolar mania. ECT, electroconvulsive therapy; IM, intramuscular.

Strength of evidence for monotherapy treatments of acute mania	
Agent	**Level of evidence**
Lithium	1
Anticonvulsant	
Valproate	1
Carbamazepine	1
Oxcarbazepine	2
Lamotrigine	1 (–ve)
Topiramate	1 (–ve)
Gabapentin	2 (–ve)
Tiagabine	3 (–ve)
Atypical antipsychotics	
Olanzapine	1
Risperidone	1
Quetiapine	1
Ziprasidone	1
Aripiprazole	1
Asenapine	1
Clozapine	3
Other treatments	
Haloperidol	1
Chlorpromazine	1
Clonazepam	2
Verapamil	2 (–ve)
ECT	3

Table 8.3 Strength of evidence for monotherapy treatments of acute mania. ECT, electroconvulsive therapy. From Yatham et al [1,3].

Strength of evidence for combination treatments of acute mania	
Agent	**Level of evidence**
Lithium/valproate + antipsychotic	1
Lithium + valproate	3
Lithium + carbamazepine	2
Valproate + carbamazepine	3
Risperidone + carbamazepine	3
Adjunctive gabapentin	2 (–ve)
Adjunctive lamotrigine	2 (–ve)
Adjunctive repetitive transcranial magnetic stimulation	3 (–ve)

Table 8.4 Strength of evidence for combination treatments of acute mania. From Yatham et al [1,3].

Drawbacks of lithium therapy include its slow onset of action, its narrow therapeutic index (recommended plasma level 0.8–1.2 mmol/L), poor tolerability – especially at higher doses – and risk of 'rebound mania' on withdrawal [8]. Despite these shortcomings, lithium is still widely used in many countries and is often seen as the gold standard comparator for newer agents.

Lithium has also been evaluated in relation to other antimanic agents. Head-to-head comparisons with antipsychotic drugs (usually chlorpromazine) have generally found lithium to be superior in terms of overall improvement in symptoms, mood, and ideation, but worse with respect to motor hyperactivity and onset of action. Moreover, lithium was as efficacious as quetiapine in a 12-week, randomized, double-blind trial [9] and comparable to aripiprazole in a similar one [10]. In a three-arm randomized study comparing placebo, lithium, and valproate, lithium and valproate were similarly effective in improving manic symptoms [11].

Randomized comparisons of a mood stabiliser (lithium or valproate) alone or in combination with antipsychotics generally found that the combinations were superior to monotherapy for the rapid control of manic symptoms [12–15], but not always [16–20]. Lithium has also been found to be well tolerated in combination with either antipsychotics or anticonvulsants [21].

Anticonvulsants

Two double-blind studies have found valproate to be superior to placebo and as effective as lithium in the treatment of acute mania [11,22]. A pooled analysis of these studies indicated that 54% of patients treated with valproate experienced a reduction of at least 50% in manic symptomatology. Unlike lithium, valproate has a rapid onset of action, producing significant clinical improvements within 1 week, and is equally effective in treating mixed and classic mania [7]. A 12-week open, randomized trial compared sodium valproate to lithium in patients with mania demonstrated comparable efficacy of both compounds with some advantages for valproate over lithium in secondary efficacy measures as well as tolerability [23].

Carbamazepine has been evaluated in two randomized, double-blind studies which used an extended-release formulation of carbamazepine as monotherapy for the acute treatment of manic or mixed episodes [24,25]. Both trials found carbamazepine to be significantly superior to placebo; side effects included dizziness, somnolence, nausea, vomiting, ataxia, blurred vision, dyspepsia, dry mouth, pruritus, and speech disorder.

Two studies have compared carbamazepine with lithium in a randomized controlled manner, with conflicting results. One found that lithium was superior [26] while the other found the drugs to be equivalent [27]. Two studies comparing carbamazepine with chlorpromazine have found no differences between the drugs. A double-blind study found that carbamazepine in combination with lithium was as effective as lithium plus haloperidol in the treatment of acute mania [28]. Another study found no advantage of adding olanzapine compared with placebo in patients taking carbamazepine [29], and similar results occured in the subgroup of patients who were on carbamazepine in a risperidone versus placebo study [18].

In all these studies, the antimanic effect of carbamazepine became evident after 1–2 weeks. Uncontrolled studies have suggested a role for carbamazepine in rapid cycling and mixed states, but these require confirmation.

There is some limited evidence that oxcarbazepine, stucturally similar to carbamazepine, may posess antimanic effects [30,31].

Newer anticonvulsants such as lamotrigine, gabapentin, and topiramate have failed to demonstrate superiority over placebo in randomized controlled studies of bipolar mania [32–34].

Typical antipsychotics

Despite the widespread use of these agents, especially in the past, placebo-controlled trial evidence showing that older antipsychotics are effective specifically in treating acute mania has only recently become available. Historically, one study reported that chlorpromazine was significantly superior to placebo on a global impression scale [35], while another found that pimozide was superior to placebo on psychotic symptoms but not mood symptoms [36]. In recent years, haloperidol has been shown to be more efficacious than placebo and at least as efficacious as atypical antipsychotics [37–41], albeit generally less tolerated [42].

Several double-blind studies have compared antipsychotics with lithium or carbamazepine, as summarized above. A meta-analysis that included many of these studies found that lithium was significantly superior to antipsychotics, with response rates of 89% and 54%, respectively [43]. However, chlorpromazine has been shown to be more effective than lithium in highly active manic patients [44], as well as having a more rapid onset of action.

Neurological side effects of standard antipsychotics seem to be more frequent in patients with bipolar disorder than in those with schizophrenia. Adverse effects include an increased risk of tardive dyskinesia when treatment is continued after remission of the acute episode. Another important issue is that typical antipsychotics may be less efficacious than lithium and than atypicals in the prevention of the switch to depression [37].

Atypical antipsychotics

Two randomized studies have found olanzapine to be significantly superior to placebo in the treatment of acute mania [45,46], and the magnitude of response was similar in patients with mixed episodes or rapid cycling [47,48].

Another randomized controlled trial showed that olanzapine was as effective as haloperidol in manic patients [37]. In addition, two randomized trials have compared olanzapine monotherapy with valproate monotherapy; one, which was probably underpowered [49], showed equivalent efficacy [50], whereas the other found olanzapine to be superior but with more side effects [51].

A study of adjunctive therapy in patients who were partially unresponsive to an initial mood stabiliser (valproate or lithium) also found that adding olanzapine was significantly more effective than adding placebo [13], but this was not the case when the mood stabiliser was carbamazepine [28]. Intramuscular injection of olanzapine reduces agitation within 2 hours [52].

The efficacy of risperidone monotherapy for the treatment of acute mania has been demonstrated in three randomized, double-blind, placebo-controlled studies [38,53,54]. Risperidone has also been studied as adjunctive treatment alongside traditional mood stabilisers (lithium or valproate) [12,18]. As mentioned above, combination therapy outperformed the mood stabiliser alone, although the addition of risperidone increased the incidence of extrapyramidal symptoms.

Ziprasidone has been evaluated as monotherapy for acute manic or mixed episodes in two large, randomized, double-blind, placebo-controlled studies [55,56]. The drug has an onset of action at day 2 and was significantly superior to placebo in both studies. Side effects included somnolence, dizziness, extrapyramidal syndrome, nausea, akathisia, and tremor. A further placebo-controlled, haloperidol-referenced trial confirmed the early onset of action of ziprasidone and the superior tolerability over haloperidol, but the latter was more efficacious at high doses [40]. In the only adjunctive ziprasidone study in mania, the study drug separated from placebo at week 1 but not at study endpoint [20].

Consistent with the other antipsychotics, aripiprazole monotherapy was shown to be superior to placebo in the acute treatment of manic or mixed episodes in two randomized controlled trials [57,58]. The clinical benefit was apparent from day 4, and side effects included nausea, dyspepsia, somnolence, vomiting, insomnia, and akathisia. A third study failed [59], but two recent studies compared aripiprazole with placebo and an active comparator, namely lithium [10] or haloperidol [41], showing superiority over placebo and similar efficacy to the comparators. Another study compared aripiprazole with haloperidol over 12 weeks; the drugs were similarly efficacious with respect to manic symptoms, but extrapyramidal side effects were more common with haloperidol [42]. When aripiprazole was investigated as adjunctive therapy in patients with partial or poor response to lithium or valproate, it outperformed placebo but there was some incidence of akathisia, especially in patients on lithium [15]. For this and other reasons (activation), it is recommended to start aripiprazole therapy at a moderate dose and to add a benzodiazepine during the first few weeks [60].

The efficacy of quetiapine in acute mania has been compared with lithium and haloperidol in separate, randomized, double-blind studies [9,39], which also had a placebo arm. Quetiapine was superior to placebo in both studies [61], and side effects included dry mouth, somnolence, weight gain, and dizziness. Quetiapine was also assessed as add-on therapy in patients who remained manic after at least 7 days of treatment with lithium or valproate in two trials [14,19]. In one of them, adjunctive therapy with quetiapine was associated with a significantly higher response rate and reduction in manic symptoms than with placebo [14]. The target dose of quetiapine in mania is generally around 600 mg [62].

An extended-release (XR) version of quetiapine has been studied as monotherapy in 316 patients with acute mania or mixed episodes. Compared with placebo, quetiapine XR had greater response rates and improvement in core mania symptoms. The most common side effects with quetiapine XR were sedation, dry mouth, somnolence, and headache [63].

Paliperidone extended-release has been recently studied as monotherapy in mania in a three-arm, placebo- and quetiapine-controlled trial, in which paliperidone 3–12 mg/day and quetiapine 400–800 mg/day were superior to placebo over a 3-week period. In a 9-week extension period, which did not include the placebo arm, paliperidone extended-release was noninferior to quetiapine [64].

Asenapine was approved in the United States in 2009 and in Europe in 2010. In a 3-week study, it had superior efficacy in acute mania compared with placebo and was noninferior to olanzapine [65,66]. The noninferiority of asenapine versus olanzapine was confirmed in a 9-week, double-blind extension study. [67]. In these trials, asenapine was well tolerated; side effects included sedation, dizziness, insomnia, headache, and somnolence [65–67]. Another placebo-controlled study assessed the efficacy and safety of adjunctive asenapine in patients with acute mania or mixed episodes who had not responded to lithium or valproate. After 12 weeks, significant improvement was seen in the asenapine group versus the placebo group [68].

Amisulpride has not been studied in double-blind, placebo-controlled designs, but a small study suggested that, similar to other atypical antipsychotics, it is effective in the treatment of acute mania [69]. In an open, randomized trial, amisulpride combined with valproate was better tolerated and as effective as haloperidol in combination with valproate [70].

The prototype, atypical, antipsychotic drug clozapine has not been evaluated in the treatment of acute bipolar mania in a double-blind, controlled study. Nevertheless, several open trials suggest that clozapine is effective in this setting, including in patients with mixed mania or a history of rapid cycling, and clozapine is often reserved for use in highly refractory cases.

Figures 8.1 and 8.2 summarize the monotherapy and adjunctive placebo-controlled trials of second-generation antipsychotics in acute mania. All this growing evidence on the efficacy of both monotherapy and

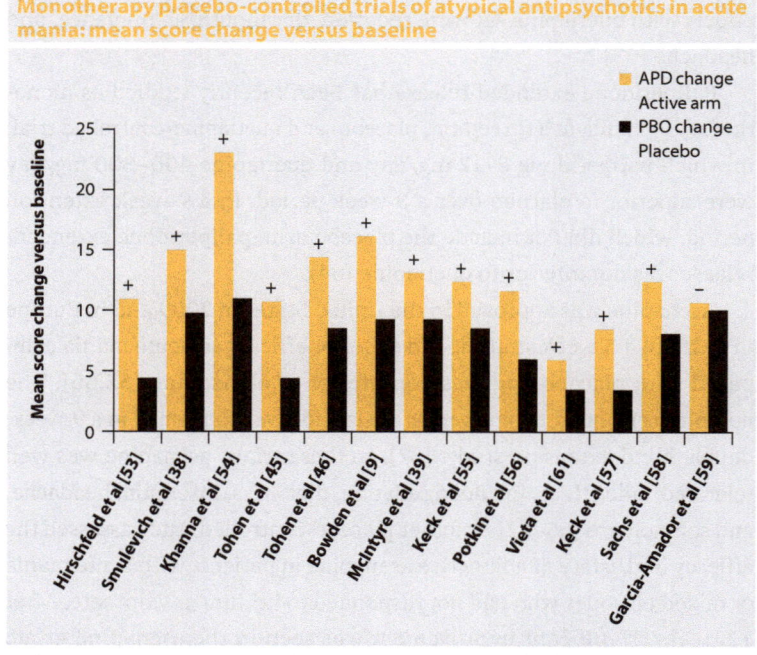

Figure 8.1. Monotherapy placebo-controlled trials of atypical antipsychotics in acute mania: mean score change versus baseline. APD, antipsychotic drug; PBO, placebo; +, statistical significance on the primary outcome.

combination therapy of atypical antipsychotics with or without lithium or valproate (but not carbamazepine) suggests that, in clinical practice, the decision to use only an atypical or a combination of an atypical and a mood stabiliser should rely on the previous course of illness, the severity of the current episode, and issues related to tolerability. In general, combination is the rule rather than the exception [71].

Benzodiazepines

Several randomized controlled trials have found lorazepam or clonazepam to be as effective as lithium or superior to placebo in the treatment of mania, but these trials were biased by the concomitant use of antipsychotics. However, a small double-blind study of benzodiazepine monotherapy found that lorazepam was superior to clonazepam, with 39.5% and 0% of patients achieving remission, respectively [72].

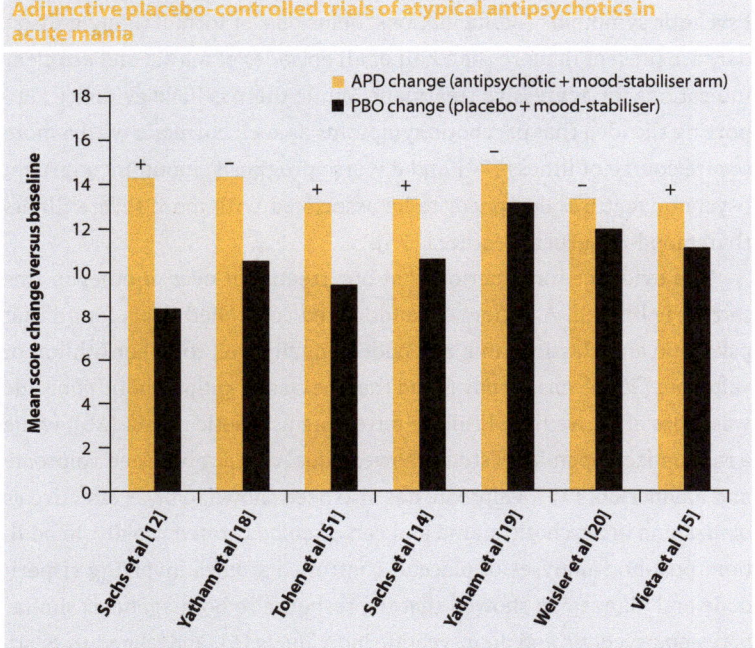

Figure 8.2 Adjunctive placebo-controlled trials of atypical antipsychotics in acute mania.
APD, antipsychotic drug; PBO, placebo; +, statistical significance on the primary outcome.

In a randomized comparison of adjunctive intramuscular clonazepam versus haloperidol in agitated psychotic manic patients, symptoms were reduced more rapidly by haloperidol, although there was no difference between the groups after 2 hours [73].

Benzodiazepines are often used as adjuncts to lithium, anticonvulsants, or antipsychotics, for the treatment of symptoms such as agitation, anxiety, or insomnia. Some drugs that have little sedative effects (ziprasidone, aripiprazole) may be more tolerable within the first days of therapy in conjunction with benzodiazepines.

Potential disadvantages of the use of benzodiazepines include the risk of dependence and the possible induction of either dysphoria or disinhibition. These drugs should be withdrawn once the manic symptoms have begun to subside.

Psychotic symptoms

Psychotic symptoms (hallucinations, delusions, or formal thought disorder) are present in more than half of all episodes of mania and are clear indications for aggressive treatment. While there is little evidence supporting the idea that psychotic symptoms as such correlate with a more severe course of illness [74] and a worse prognosis, mood-incongruent psychotic features do appear to be associated with more severe illness than mood-congruent features [75].

The evidence for superiority of one treatment over another in this setting is limited. A review of randomized controlled trials found that psychotic and classic mania responded equally well to either lithium or valproate [76]. A small study found that the classic antipsychotic pimozide was more effective than lithium in treating psychotic mania [36], while a randomized open-label study showed equal efficacy between valproate and haloperidol [77]. Valproate has also been shown to be as effective as olanzapine in psychotic mania and can often be titrated rapidly. In addition, post-hoc analyses of placebo-controlled studies involving risperidone and olanzapine showed that the response to both agents is similar between psychotic and nonpsychotic individuals [5], and a head-to-head, randomized controlled trial in nonpsychotic manic patients showed no significant differences between the two drugs in terms of efficacy [78].

Clinical guidelines also vary in their recommendations for first-line treatment of psychotic mania. Some favor anticonvulsants over lithium when psychotic symptoms are present, while others recommend the combination of a mood stabiliser (valproate or lithium) plus an antipsychotic. Both US and British guidelines favor the use of atypical antipsychotic drugs over traditional antipsychotics in view of their generally better tolerability. with regards to neurological side effects, but some other guidelines such as the Texas Medication Algorithms give preference to drugs with low extrapyramidal side effects but also low metabolic risk [79].

Acute episodes in children and adolescents

There is a growing body of evidence from randomized controlled trials indicating that childhood- and adolescent-onset bipolar disorder will respond to the same agents as adult-onset illness [80].

Lithium has demonstrated superior efficacy over placebo in the acute treatment of children and adolescents with bipolar disorder and comorbid substance abuse [81]. Lithium has also been found to be effective in treating manic or mixed episodes in several open trials, and was effective in combination with an anticonvulsant in a retrospective study [82].

In prospective open studies, valproate was an effective treatment in children and adolescents with bipolar disorder [83,84]. Most of the evidence concerns the treatment of mania but there is also some experience with long-term treatment [85].

A randomized comparison of valproate alone or in combination with quetiapine found that the combination was significantly more effective than monotherapy in treating acute mania in adolescents [86]. A second trial suggested that quetiapine was more effective than valproate in adolescents with mania [87]. A trial of oxcarbazepine failed to beat placebo in children and adolescents [88]. Finally, a randomized, placebo-controlled trial showed that olanzapine was superior to placebo in acutely manic adolescents [89], and recent positive placebo-controlled trials have also been conducted with risperidone and with aripiprazole [90,91].

The American Academy of Child and Adolescent Psychiatry has specific guidelines on the management of pediatric bipolar disorder; these were last updated in 2005 [92]. A related practice parameter was published in January 2007 [93].

Long-term maintenance therapy

Maintenance medication is generally recommended following a single acute manic episode, in view of the 95% lifetime risk of recurrence. Maintenance treatment is also appropriate in patients who experience a breakthrough episode during the first year of treatment following an acute episode, and in chronically ill patients with a long cycle length who do not achieve sufficient remission of acute symptoms to be classified as 'recovered'. Psychosocial interventions are a valuable adjunct to maintenance medication and are discussed in Chapter 10.

The choice of pharmacological prophylaxis will be determined by the patient's history and response to prior treatment trials. The goals of maintenance treatment include relapse prevention, reduction of subthreshold symptoms, reduction of suicide risk, reduction in cycle frequency and mood instability, and an improvement in overall function. The most important maintenance options in bipolar mania are lithium, valproate, lamotrigine, carbamazepine, and some atypical antipsychotics, with the best evidence available so far involving quetiapine, olanzapine, and aripiprazole. A number needed to treat (NNT) analysis confirmed this evidence for lithium and the atypical antipsychotics [94].

Cost may also be a factor in determining which maintenance treatment option to use. Data from a Markov model based on available clinical data of societal and payer perspectives in the United States indicated that overall, the combination of extended-release quetiapine with either lithium or valproate may have the lowest incremental cost per quality-adjusted life year [95].

Guideline recommendations for maintenance treatment are summarized in Table 8.5 [2–4,96].

Lithium

The prophylactic efficacy of lithium in bipolar I disorder has been reported for several decades, and was confirmed in a Cochrane review [97] and two meta-analyses [98,99]. At optimal dosing, lithium reduces recurrences

	First line	Second line
Comparison of guideline recommendations for maintenance treatment of bipolar mania		
American Psychiatric Association, 2002 [2]	Lithium *or* valproate	Combination of first-line agents
	Possibly carbamazepine, lamotrigine or oxcarbazepine	ECT
	Continue the treatment	Antipsychotics should be discontinued
World Federation of Societies of Biological Psychiatry, 2004 [96]	Lithium, olanzapine, other atypical antipsychotics	Risperidone (add-on)
		Psychotherapy
		ECT
Canadian Network for Mood and Anxiety Disorders (CANMAT) and International Society for Bipolar Disorders (ISBD), 2009 [3]	Lithium, aripiprazole, olanzapine, adjunctive risperidone, adjunctive ziprasidone	Risperidone (add-on), carbamazepine, combination of first-line agents
		Psychotherapy
British Association for Psychopharmacology, 2009 [4]	Lithium, aripiprazole, olanzapine, quetiapine, valproate	Carbamazepine, combination therapy
		Psychotherapy

Table 8.5 Comparison of guideline recommendations for maintenance treatment of bipolar mania. ECT, electroconvulsive therapy.

by around 50%, and appears to be more effective against manic than depressive relapses [100–102]. Moreover, lithium may have antisuicidal effects independently from its efficacy in preventing recurrences [103].

However, the efficacy of lithium in clinical practice may be less than that in controlled clinical trials, in part due to comorbidity and poor adherence. Therefore, putative predictors of a favorable response to lithium (eg, family history of bipolar disorder, no rapid cycling, complete interepisode recovery, no substance abuse, good adherence) should also be considered [104]. Indeed, the increased risk of relapse after sudden discontinuation of lithium, and the potential for a lack of response when lithium is reintroduced, have led some experts to advise against using lithium in patients judged unwilling or unlikely to adhere to treatment for at least 2 years [8].

Anticonvulsants

Despite high expectations for the prophylactic efficacy of valproate, the agent failed to demonstrate superiority over placebo in preventing recurrence of bipolar episodes in a randomized controlled trial [105]. However, in randomized studies with active comparators, valproate was equivalent to lithium [106] and olanzapine [107] in the prevention of bipolar recurrence. The BALANCE study found that the combination of lithium plus valproate was statistically superior to valproate monotherapy and slightly superior to lithium monotherapy for the prevention of new manic episodes [108].

Carbamazepine is widely used in patients who have failed treatment with lithium, especially in Europe and Japan. It has been shown to be superior to placebo in a small trial [109], and was equal to lithium in a meta-analysis [110]. However, the studies were too heterogeneous to allow conclusive results. In a 2.5-year randomized study of lithium and carbamazepine, lithium was associated with a lower overall rate of relapse (28% versus 47%) and fewer adverse events [111]. However, carbamazepine appeared more effective than lithium in patients with atypical features such as mixed states and delusions [112], suggesting that it has a broader spectrum of activity. A study of treatment-naïve bipolar disorder patients showed that lithium was slightly more effective than carbamazepine in preventing relapses over a 2-year period, although carbamazepine was superior during the first 6 months [113].

Limited controlled data are available on the long-term outcome of bipolar disorder patients treated with oxcarbazepine [30,31], but results from one study suggest that it might have some prophylactic efficacy, especially on impulsivity [114].

A pilot, randomized, placebo-controlled trial suggested that gabapentin might have some prophylactic effects when used in conjunction with lithium in euthymic patients with a highly recurring course [115].

Antipsychotics

Olanzapine has demonstrated long-term efficacy in randomized controlled trials. Compared with placebo, olanzapine significantly reduced rates of new manic and depressive relapses, with the effect most pronounced for manic relapses [116]. Similar results were found when patients were given olanzapine long-term after they had responded to olanzapine for acute bipolar disorder [117].

In a 1-year, randomized, double-blind study, olanzapine was superior to lithium in reducing recurrent manic and mixed episodes [118]. Olanzapine was also associated with significantly fewer discontinuations due to side effects. In a 47-week, double-blind study comparing olanzapine and valproate for manic or mixed episodes, the median time to remission was shorter for olanzapine than for valproate, although overall remission rates were similar [107].

Another atypical antipsychotic, aripiprazole, was compared with placebo in a 6-month, randomized controlled study [119]. Active therapy significantly prolonged the time to recurrence and reduced the number of mood episodes versus placebo. The results were sustained at the 100-week, double-blind, follow-up extension [120]. Subgroup analysis indicated that aripiprazole was superior to placebo in preventing manic, but not depressive, episodes.

Quetiapine has recently confirmed its efficacy in the long-term treatment of bipolar disorder as anticipated in several pilot studies [121,122], with comparably positive results in the prevention of manic and depressive recurrences, irrespective of the polarity of the index episode [123,124]. Those studies indicate that quetiapine, when prescribed in combination with lithium or valproate, works as a mood stabiliser but can also cause some weight gain and glucose increase. A recent monotherapy study corroborated the findings of the two adjunctive long-term trials [125].

A recent randomized, double-blind, study compared adjunctive, long-acting, injectable risperidone with adjunctive placebo as maintenance therapy in patients with frequently relapsing bipolar disorder. Patients in the risperidone group had significantly longer time to relapse of any mood episode. However, the study was not powered to show efficacy for the prevention of mania and depression separately and therefore it is unclear if the drug is effective for both poles [126]. A previous open study suggested that injectable risperidone would be more effective in preventing mania than depression [127]. A 40-week extension of the 12-week adjunctive asenapine study found no difference in efficacy between asenapine and placebo, although the study drug was well tolerated [68].

In clinical practice, the use of second-generation antipsychotics as adjuncts for the long-term treatment of bipolar disorder is growing [128] and could be particularly useful in patients with manic-predominant polarity [129], at least in the case of olanzapine, aripiprazole, long-acting injectable risperidone, and ziprasidone. Quetiapine would have a more balanced profile. Table 8.6 shows proposed operational criteria for long-term treatment with atypicals. Two out of six criteria would qualify for long-term treatment with those drugs, according to guidelines of the Barcelona Bipolar Disorders Program.

Criteria for long-term treatment with atypical antipsychotics in bipolar disorder

- Patients with a recent severe, psychotic, manic episode
- Patients with a history of relapse after discontinuation of antipsychotic medication
- Patients with manic-predominant polarity
- Patients partially or fully refractory to conventional mood stabilizers
- Rapid cyclers
- Patients showing excellent tolerability to atypical antipsychotics

Table 8.6 Criteria for long-term treatment with atypical antipsychotics in bipolar disorder.

References

1   Yatham LN, Kennedy SH, O'Donovan C; Canadian Network for Mood and Anxiety Treatments. Canadian Network for Mood and Anxiety Treatments (CANMAT) guidelines for the management of patients with bipolar disorder: consensus and controversies. *Bipolar Disord*. 2005;7(suppl 3):5-69.

2   Fountoulakis KN, Vieta E, Sanchez-Moreno J, et al. Treatment guidelines for bipolar disorder: a critical review. *J Affect Disord*. 2005;86:1-10.

3   Yatham LN, Kennedy SH, Schaffer A, et al. Canadian Network for Mood and Anxiety Treatments (CANMAT) and International Society for Bipolar Disorders (ISBD) collaborative update of CANMAT guidelines for the management of patients with bipolar disorder: update 2009. Bipolar Disord 2009; 11:225-255.

4   Goodwin GM; Consensus Group of the British Association for Psychopharmacology. Evidence-based guidelines for treating bipolar disorder: revised second edition— recommendations from the British Association for Psychopharmacology. *J Psychopharmacol*. 2009;23:346-388.

5   Grunze H, Vieta E, Goodwin GM, et al. WFSBP Task Force on Treatment Guidelines for Bipolar Disorders. The World Federation of Societies of Biological Psychiatry (WFSBP) guidelines for the biological treatment of bipolar disorders.: update 2009 on the treatment of acute mania. *World J Biol Psychiatry*. 2009;10:85-116.

6   Bowden CL. Key treatment studies of lithium in manic-depressive illness: efficacy and side effects. *J Clin Psychiatry*. 1998;59(suppl 6):13-19.

7   Swann AC, Bowden CL, Morris D, et al. Depression during mania. Treatment response to lithium or divalproex. *Arch Gen Psychiatry*. 1997;54:37-42.

8   Goodwin GM. Recurrence of mania after lithium withdrawal. Implications for the use of lithium in the treatment of bipolar affective disorder. *Br J Psychiatry*. 1994;164:52.

9   Bowden CL, Grunze H, Mullen J, et al. A randomized, double-blind, placebo-controlled efficacy and safety study of quetiapine or lithium as monotherapy for mania in bipolar disorder. *J Clin Psychiatry*. 2005;66:111-121.

10   Keck PE, Orsulak PJ, Cutler AJ, et al; the CN-138-35 Study Group. Aripiprazole monotherapy in the treatment of acute bipolar I mania: a randomized, double-blind, placebo- and lithium-controlled study. *J Affect Disord*. 2009;112:36-49.

11   Bowden CL, Brugger AM, Swann AC, et al. Efficacy of divalproex versus lithium and placebo in the treatment of mania. *JAMA*. 1994;271:918-924.

12   Sachs GS, Grossman F, Ghaemi SN, et al. Combination of a mood stabilizer with risperidone or haloperidol for treatment of acute mania: a double-blind, placebo-controlled comparison of efficacy and safety. *Am J Psychiatry*. 2002;159:1146-1154.

13   Tohen M, Chengappa KN, Suppes T, et al. Efficacy of olanzapine in combination with valproate or lithium in the treatment of mania in patients partially nonresponsive to valproate or lithium monotherapy. *Arch Gen Psychiatry*. 2002;59:62-69.

14   Sachs G, Chengappa KN, Suppes T et al. Quetiapine with lithium or divalproex for the treatment of bipolar mania: a randomized, double-blind, placebo-controlled study. *Bipolar Disord*. 2004; 6:213-223.

15   Vieta E, T'joen C, McQuade RD et al. Efficacy of adjunctive aripiprazole to either valproate or lithium in bipolar mania patients partially nonresponsive to valproate/lithium monotherapy: a placebo-controlled study. *Am J Psychiatry*. 2008; 165:1316-1325.

16   Garfinkel PE, Stancer HC, Persad E. A comparison of haloperidol, lithium carbonate, and their combination in the treatment of mania. *J Affect Disord*. 1980;2:279-288.

17   Johnstone EC, Crow TJ, Frith CD, et al. The Northwick Park 'functional' psychosis study: diagnosis and treatment response. *Lancet*. 1988;2:119-125.

18   Yatham LN, Grossman F, Augustyns I, et al. Mood stabilisers plus risperidone or placebo in the treatment of acute mania: international, double-blind, randomised controlled trial. *Br J Psychiatry*. 2003;182:141-147.

19   Yatham LN, Vieta E, Young AH, et al. A double blind, randomized, placebo-controlled trial of quetiapine as an add-on therapy to lithium or divalproex for the treatment of bipolar mania. *Int Clin Psychopharmacol*. 2007; 22:212-220.

20   Weisler R, Dunn J, English P. Ziprasidone in adjunctive treatment of acute bipolar mania: randomized, double-blind, placebo-controlled trial. 16th European College of Neuropsychopharmachology Congress, Prague, Czech Republic, September 20–24, 2003.

21   Freeman MP, Stoll AL. Mood stabilizer combinations: a review of safety and efficacy. *Am J Psychiatry*. 1998;155:12-21.

22   Pope HG Jr, McElroy SL, Keck PE, et al. Valproate in treatment of acute mania. A placebo controlled study. *Arch Gen Psychiatry*. 1991;48:62-68.

23   Bowden C, Gögüs A, Grunze H, et al. A 12-week, open, randomized trial comparing sodium valproate to lithium in patients with bipolar I disorder suffering from a manic episode. *Int Clin Psychopharmacol*. 2008; 23:254-262.

24   Weisler RH, Kalali AH, Ketter TA. A multicenter, randomized, double-blind, placebo-controlled trial of extended-release carbamazepine capsules as monotherapy for bipolar disorder patients with manic or mixed episodes. *J Clin Psychiatry*. 2004;65:478-484.

25   Weisler RH, Keck PE Jr, Swann AC, et al. Extended-release carbamazepine capsules as monotherapy for acute mania in bipolar disorder: a multicenter, randomized, double-blind, placebo-controlled trial. *J Clin Psychiatry*. 2005;66:323-330.

26   Lerer B, Moore N, Meyendorff E, et al. Carbamazepine versus lithium in mania: a double-blind study. *J Clin Psychiatry*. 1987;48:89-93.

27   Small JG, Klapper MH, Milstein V, et al. Carbamazepine compared with lithium in the treatment of mania. *Arch Gen Psychiatry*. 1991;48:915-921.

28   Small JG, Klapper MH, Marhenke JD, et al. Lithium combined with carbamazepine or haloperidol in the treatment of mania. *Psychopharmacol Bull*. 1995;31:265-272.

29   Tohen M, Bowden CL, Smulevich AB, et al. Olanzapine plus carbamazepine v. carbamazepine alone in treating manic episodes. *Br J Psychiatry*. 2008;192:135-143.

30   Vieta E. The role of third-generation anticonvulsants in the treatment of bipolar disorder. *Clin Neuropsychiatry*. 2004;1:159-164.

31   Popova E, Leighton C, Bernabarre A, et al. Oxcarbazepine in the treatment of bipolar and schizoaffective disorders. *Expert Rev Neurother*. 2007;7:617-626.

32   Goldsmith DR, Wagstaff AJ, Ibbotson T, et al. Lamotrigine: a review of its use in bipolar disorder. *Drugs*. 2003;63:2029-2050.

33   Pande AC, Crockatt JG, Janney CA, et al. Gabapentin in bipolar disorder: a placebo-controlled trial of adjunctive therapy. Gabapentin Bipolar Disorder Study Group. *Bipolar Disord*. 2000;2(3 Pt 2):249-255.

34   Kushner SF, Khan A, Lane R, et al. Topiramate monotherapy in the management of acute mania: results of four double-blind placebo-controlled trials. *Bipolar Disord*. 2006;8:15-27.

35   Klein DF, Oaks G. Importance of psychiatric diagnosis in prediction of clinical drug effect. *Arch Gen Psychiatry*. 1967;16:118-126.

36   Johnstone EC, Crow TJ, Frith CD, et al. The Northwick Park 'functional' psychosis study: diagnosis and treatment response. *Lancet*. 1988;2:119-125.

37   Tohen M, Goldberg JF, Gonzalez-Pinto Arrillaga AM, et al. A 12-week, double-blind comparison of olanzapine vs haloperidol in the treatment of acute mania. *Arch Gen Psychiatry*. 2003;60:1218-1226.

38   Smulevich AB, Khanna S, Eerdekens M, et al. Acute and continuation risperidone monotherapy in bipolar mania: a 3-week placebocontrolled trial followed by a 9-week double-blind trial of risperidone and haloperidol. *Eur Neuropsychopharmacol*. 2005;15:75-84.

39   McIntyre RS, Brecher M, Paulsson B, et al. Quetiapine or haloperidol as monotherapy for bipolar mania: a 12-week, double-blind, randomised, parallel-group, placebo-controlled trial. *Eur Neuropsychopharmacol*. 2005;15:573-585.

40   Vieta E, Ramey T, Keller D, et al. Ziprasidone in the treatment of acute mania: 12-week placebo-controlled, haloperidol-referenced study. *J Psychopharmacol*. 2010;24:547-558.

41   Young AH, Oren DA, Lowy A, et al. Aripiprazole monotherapy in acute mania: 12-week, randomised placebo- and haloperidol-controlled study. *Br J Psychiatry*. 2009;194:40-48.

42   Vieta E, Bourin M, Sanchez R, et al. Effectiveness of aripiprazole versus haloperidol in acute bipolar mania: double-blind, randomised, comparative 12-week trial. *Br J Psychiatry*. 2005;187:235-242.

43   Janicak PG, Newman RH, Davis JM. Advances in the treatment of mania and related disorders: a reappraisal. *Psychiatr Ann*. 1992;22:92-103.

44   Prien RF, Caffey EM, Klett CJ. Comparison of lithium carbonate and chlorpromazine in the treatment of mania. *Arch Gen Psychiatry*. 1972;26:146-153.

45   Tohen M, Sanger TM, McElroy SL, et al. Olanzapine versus placebo in the treatment of acute mania. *Am J Psychiatry*. 1999;15:702-709.

46   Tohen M, Jacobs TG, Grundy SL, et al. Efficacy of olanzapine in acute bipolar mania: a double-blind, placebo-controlled study. *Arch Gen Psychiatry*. 2000;57:841-849.

47   Baldessarini RJ, Hennen J, Wilson M, et al. Olanzapine versus placebo in acute mania: treatment responses in subgroups. *J Clin Psychopharmacol*. 2003;23:370-376.

48   Sanger TM, Tohen M, Vieta E, et al. Olanzapine in the acute treatment of bipolar I disorder with a history of rapid cycling. *J Affect Disord*. 2003;73:155-161.

49   Vieta E. Divalproex versus olanzapine in mania. *J Clin Psychiatry*. 2003;64:1266.

50   Zajecka JM, Weisler R, Sachs G, et al. A comparison of the efficacy, safety, and tolerability of divalproex sodium and olanzapine in the treatment of bipolar disorder. *J Clin Psychiatry*. 2002;63:1148-1155.

51   Tohen M, Baker RW, Altshuler LL, et al. Olanzapine versus divalproex in the treatment of acute mania. *Am J Psychiatry*. 2002;159:1011-1017.

52   Meehan K, Zhang F, David S, et al. A double-blind, randomized comparison of the efficacy and safety of intramuscular injections of olanzapine, lorazepam, or placebo in treating acutely agitated patients diagnosed with bipolar mania. *J Clin Psychopharmacol.* 2001;21:389-397.

53   Hirschfeld RM, Keck PE Jr, Kramer M, et al. Rapid antimanic effect of risperidone monotherapy: a 3-week multicenter, double-blind, placebo-controlled trial. *Am J Psychiatry.* 2004;161:1057-1065.

54   Khanna S, Vieta E, Lyons B, et al. Risperidone in the treatment of acute bipolar mania: double-blind, placebo-controlled study. *Br J Psychiatry.* 2005;187:229-234.

55   Keck PE Jr, Versiani M, Potkin S, et al; Zipradisone in Mania Study Group. Ziprasidone in the treatment of acute bipolar mania: a three-week, placebo-controlled, double-blind, randomized trial. *Am J Psychiatry.* 2003;160:741-748.

56   Potkin SG, Keck PE Jr, Segal S, et al. Ziprasidone in acute bipolar mania: a 21-day randomized, double-blind, placebo-controlled replication trial. *J Clin Psychopharmacol.* 2005;25:301-310.

57   Keck PE Jr, Marcus R, Tourkodimitris S, et al. A placebo-controlled, double-blind study of the efficacy and safety of aripiprazole in patients with acute bipolar mania. *Am J Psychiatry.* 2003;160:1651-1658.

58   Sachs G, Sanchez R, Marcus R, et al. Aripiprazole in the treatment of acute manic or mixed episodes in patients with bipolar I disorder: a 3-week placebo-controlled study. *J Psychopharmacol.* 2006;20:536-546.

59   García-Amador M, Pacchiarotti I, Valentí M et al. Role of aripiprazole in treating mood disorders. *Expert Rev Neurother.* 2006;6:1777-1783.

60   Vieta E, Franco C. Advances in the treatment of mania: aripiprazole. *Actas Esp Psiquiatr.* 2008;36:158-164.

61   Vieta E, Mullen J, Brecher M, et al. Quetiapine monotherapy for mania associated with bipolar disorder: combined analysis of two international, double-blind, randomised, placebo-controlled studies. *Curr Med Res Opin.* 2005;21:923-934.

62   Vieta E, Goldberg JF, Mullen J, et al. Quetiapine in the treatment of acute mania: target dose for efficacious treatment. *J Affect Disord.* 2007;100(suppl 1):S23-S31.

63   Cutler AJ, Datto C, Nordenhem A, et al. Extended-release quetiapine as monotherapy for the treatment of adults with acute mania: a randomized, double-blind, 3-week trial. *Clin Ther.* 2011;33:1643-1658.

64   Vieta E, Nuamah IF, Lim P. A randomized, placebo- and active-controlled study of paliperidone extended release for the treatment of acute manic and mixed episodes of bipolar I disorder. *Bipolar Disord.* 2010;12:230-243.

65   McIntyre RS, Cohen M, Zhao J, et al. A 3-week randomized, placebo-controlled trial of asenapine in the treatment of acute mania in bipolar mania and mixed states. *Bipolar Disord.* 2009;11:673-686.

66   McIntyre RS, Cohen M, Zhao J, et al. Asenapine in the treatment of acute mania in bipolar I disorder: a randomized, double-blind, placebo-controlled trial. *J Affect Disord.* 2010;122:27-38.

67   McIntyre RS, Cohen M, Zhao J, et al. Asenapine versus olanzapine in acute mania: a double-blind extension study. *Bipolar Disord.* 2009;11:815-826.

68   Szegedi A, Calabrese JR, Stet L, et al; the Apollo Study Group. Asenapine as adjunctive treatment for acute mania associated with bipolar disorder: results of a 12-week core study and 40-week extension. *J Clin Psychopharmacol.* 2012;32:46-55.

69   Vieta E, Ros S, Goikolea JM, et al. An open-label study of amisulpride in the treatment of mania. *J Clin Psychiatry.* 2005;66:575-578.

70   Thomas P, Vieta E; for the SOLMANIA study group. Amisulpride plus valproate vs haloperidol plus valproate in the treatment of acute mania of bipolar I patients: a multicenter, open-label, randomized, comparative trial. *Neuropsychiatr Dis Treat.* 2008; 4:675-686.

71   Vieta E, Panicali F, Goetz I, et al; EMBLEM Advisory Board. Olanzapine monotherapy and olanzapine combination therapy in the treatment of mania: 12-week results from the European Mania in Bipolar Longitudinal Evaluation of Medication (EMBLEM) observational study. *J Affect Disord*. 2008;106:63-72.

72   Bradwejn J, Shriqui C, Koszycki D, et al. Double-blind comparison of the effects of clonazepam and lorazepam in acute mania. *J Clin Psychopharmacol*. 1990;10:403-408.

73   Chouinard G, Annabel L, Turnier L, et al. A double-blind randomized clinical trial of rapid tranquilization with i.m. clonazepam and i.m. haloperidol in agitated psychotic patients with manic symptoms. *Can J Psychiatry*. 1993;38:S114-S121.

74   Vieta E, Phillips ML. Deconstructing bipolar disorder: a critical review of its diagnostic validity and a proposal for DSM-V and ICD-11. *Schizophr Bull*. 2007;33:886-892.

75   Toni C, Perugi G, Mata B, et al. Is mood-incongruent manic psychosis a distinct subtype? *Eur Arch Psychiatry Clin Neurosci*. 2001;251:12-17.

76   Swann A, Bowden C, Calabrese J, et al. Pattern of response to divalproex, lithium, or placebo in four naturalistic subtypes of mania. *Neuropsychopharmacology*. 2002;26:530-536.

77   McElroy SL, Keck PE, Stanton SP, et al. A randomized comparison of divalproex oral loading versus haloperidol in the initial treatment of acute psychotic mania. *J Clin Psychiatry*. 1996;57:142-146.

78   Perlis RH, Baker RW, Zarate CA Jr, et al. Olanzapine versus risperidone in the treatment of manic or mixed states in bipolar I disorder: a randomized, double-blind trial. *J Clin Psychiatry*. 2006;67:1747-1753.

79   Suppes T, Dennehy EB, Hirschfeld RM, et al; Texas Consensus Conference Panel on Medication Treatment of Bipolar Disorder. The Texas implementation of medication algorithms: update to the algorithms for treatment of bipolar I disorder. *J Clin Psychiatry*. 2005;66:870-886.

80   Weller E, Danielyan A, Weller R. Somatic treatment of bipolar disorder in children and adolescents. *Psychiatr Clin North Am*. 2004;27:155-178.

81   Geller B, Cooper T, Sun K, et al. Double-blind and placebo- controlled study of lithium for adolescent bipolar disorders with secondary substance dependency. *J Am Acad Child Adolesc Psychiatry*. 1998;37:171-178.

82   Rajeev J, Srinath S, Girimaji S, et al. A systematic chart review of the naturalistic course and treatment of early-onset bipolar disorder in a child and adolescent psychiatry center. *Compr Psychiatry*. 2004;45:148-154.

83   Kowatch R, Suppes T, Carmody T, et al. Effect size of lithium, divalproex sodium, and carbamazepine in children and adolescents with bipolar disorder. *J Am Acad Child Adolesc Psychiatry*. 2000;39:713-720.

84   Wagner K, Weller E, Carlson G, et al. An open-label trial of divalproex in children and adolescents with bipolar disorder. *J Am Acad Child Adolesc Psychiatry*. 2002;41:1224-1230.

85   Azorin JM, Findling RL. Valproate use in children and adolescents with bipolar disorder. *CNS Drugs*. 2007;21:1019-1033.

86   DelBello M, Schwiers M, Rosenberg H, et al. A double-blind, randomized, placebo-controlled study of quetiapine as adjunctive treatment for adolescent mania. *J Am Acad Child Adolesc Psychiatry*. 2002; 41:1216-1223.

87   DeBello MP, Kowatch RA, Adler CM, et al. A double-blind randomized pilot study comparing quetiapine and divalproex for adolescent mania. *J Am Acad Child Adolesc Psychiatry*. 2006;45:305-313.

88   Wagner KD, Kowatch RA, Emslie GJ et al. A double-blind, randomized, placebo-controlled trial of oxcarbazepine in the treatment of bipolar disorder in children and adolescents. *Am J Psychiatry*. 2006;163:1179-1186.

89   Tohen M, Kryzhanovskaya L, Carlson G, et al. Olanzapine versus placebo in the treatment of adolescents with bipolar mania. *Am J Psychiatry*. 2007;164:1547-1556.

90 Haas M, DelBello MP, Pandina G, et al. Risperidone for the treatment of acute mania in children and adolescents with bipolar disorder: a randomized, double-blind, placebo-controlled study. *Bipolar Disord.* 2009;11:687-700.

91 Sajatovic M, Coconcea N, Ignacio RV, et al. Aripiprazole therapy in 20 older adults with bipolar disorder: a 12-week, open-label trial. *J Clin Psychiatry.* 2008;69:41-46.

92 Kowatch RA, Fristad M, Birmaher B, et al. Treatment guidelines for children and adolescents with bipolar disorder. *J Am Acad Child Adolesc Psychiatry.* 2005;44:213-235.

93 McClellan J, Kowatch R, Findling RL, et al; Work Group on Quality Issues. Practice parameter for the assessment and treatment of children and adolescents with bipolar disorder. *J Am Acad Child Adolesc Psychiatry.* 2007;46:107-125.

94 Popovic D, Reinares M, Amann B, et al. Number needed to treat analyses of drugs used for maintenance treatment of bipolar disorder. *Psychopharmacology (Berl).* 2011;213:657-667.

95 Woodward TC, Tafesse E, Quon P, et al. Cost effectiveness of adjunctive quetiapine fumarate extended-release tablets with mood stabilizers in the maintenance treatment of bipolar I disorder. *Pharmacoeconomics.* 2010;28:751-764.

96 Grunze H, Kasper S, Goodwin G, et al. WFSBP Task Force on Treatment Guidelines for Bipolar Disorders. The World Federation of Societies of Biological Psychiatry (WFSBP) guidelines for the biological treatment of bipolar disorders. Part III: maintenance treatment. *World J Biol Psychiatry.* 2004;5:120-135.

97 Burgess S, Geddes J, Hawton K, et al. Lithium for maintenance treatment of mood disorders. *Cochrane Database Syst Rev.* 2001;(3):CD003013.

98 Davis JM, Janicak PG, Hogan DM. Mood stabilizers in the prevention of recurrent affective disorders: a meta-analysis. *Acta Psychiatr Scand.* 1999;100:406-417.

99 Geddes JR, Burgess S, Hawton K, et al. Long-term lithium therapy for bipolar disorder: systematic review and meta-analysis of randomized controlled trials. *Am J Psychiatry.* 2004;161:217-222.

100 Calabrese J, Bowden C, Sachs G, et al. A placebo-controlled 18-month trial of lamotrigine and lithium maintenance treatment in recently depressed patients with bipolar I disorder. *J Clin Psychiatry.* 2003;64:1013-1024.

101 Bowden C, Calabrese J, Sachs G, et al. A placebo-controlled 18-month trial of lamotrigine and lithium maintenance treatment in recently manic or hypomanic patients with bipolar I disorder. *Arch Gen Psychiatry.* 2003;60:392-400.

102 Nivoli AMA, Murru A, Vieta E. Lithium: still a cornerstone in the long-term treatment of bipolar disorder? *Neuropsychobiology.* 2010; 62:27-35.

103 Goodwin FK, Fireman B, Simon GE, et al. Suicide risk in bipolar disorder during treatment with lithium and divalproex. *JAMA.* 2003;290:1467-1473.

104 Abou-Saleh MT, Coppen A. Who responds to prophylactic lithium? *J Affect Disord.* 1986;10:115-125.

105 Bowden C, Calabrese J, McElroy S, et al. A randomized, placebo-controlled 12-month trial of divalproex and lithium in treatment of outpatients with bipolar I disorder. Divalproex Maintenance Study Group. *Arch Gen Psychiatry.* 2000;57:481-489.

106 Calabrese J, Shelton M, Rapport D, et al. A 20-month, double-blind, maintenance trial of lithium versus divalproex in rapid-cycling bipolar disorder. *Am J Psychiatry.* 2005;162:2152-2161.

107 Tohen M, Ketter T, Zarate C, et al. Olanzapine versus divalproex sodium for the treatment of acute mania and maintenance of remission: a 47-week study. *Am J Psychiatry.* 2003;160:1263-1271.

108 The BALANCE Investigators and Collaborators. Lithium plus valproate combination therapy versus monotherapy for relapse presentation in bipolar I disorder (BALANCE): a randomised open-label trial. *Lancet.* 2010;375:385-395.

109 Okuma T, Inanaga K, Otsuki S, et al. A preliminary double-blind study on the efficacy of carbamazepine in prophylaxis of manic-depressive illness. *Psychopharmacology (Berl)*. 1981;73:95-96.

110 Dardennes R, Even C, Bange F, et al. Comparison of carbamazepine and lithium in the prophylaxis of bipolar disorders. A meta-analysis. *Br J Psychiatry*. 1995;166:378-381.

111 Greil W, Ludwig-Mayerhofer W, Erazo N, et al. Lithium versus carbamazepine in the maintenance treatment of bipolar disorders-a randomised study. *J Affective Disord*. 1997;43:151-161.

112 Greil W, Kleindienst N, Erazo N, et al. Differential response to lithium and carbamazepine in the prophylaxis of bipolar disorder. *J Clin Psychopharmacol*. 1998;18:455-460.

113 Hartong EG, Moleman P, Hoogduin CA, et al. Prophylactic efficacy of lithium versus carbamazepine in treatment-naive bipolar patients. *J Clin Psychiatry*. 2003;64:144-151.

114 Vieta E, Cruz N, García-Campayo J, et al. A double-blind, randomized, placebo-controlled prophylaxis trial of oxcarbazepine as adjunctive treatment to lithium in the long-term treatment of bipolar I and II disorder. *Int J Neuropsychopharmacol*. 2008;11:445-452.

115 Vieta E, Manuel Goikolea J, Martinez-Aran A, et al. A double-blind, randomized, placebo-controlled, prophylaxis study of adjunctive gabapentin for bipolar disorder. *J Clin Psychiatry*. 2006;67:473-477.

116 Tohen M, Bowden C, Calabrese J, et al. Olanzapine's efficacy for relapse prevention in bipolar disorder: A randomized double-blind controlled 12-month clinical trial. *World J Biol Psychiatry*. 2004;5:51.

117 Tohen M, Calabrese JR, Sachs GS, et al. Randomized, placebo-controlled trial of olanzapine as maintenance therapy in patients with bipolar I disorder responding to acute treatment with olanzapine. *Am J Psychiatry*. 2006;163:247-256.

118 Tohen M, Greil W, Calabrese JR, et al. Olanzapine versus lithium in the maintenance treatment of bipolar disorder: a 12-month, randomized, double-blind, controlled clinical trial. *Am J Psychiatry*. 2005;162:1281-1290.

119 Keck PE Jr, Calabrese JR, McQuade RD, et al. A randomized, double-blind, placebo-controlled 26-week trial of aripiprazole in recently manic patients with bipolar I disorder. *J Clin Psychiatry*. 2006;67:626-637.

120 Keck PE Jr, Calabrese JR, McIntyre RS, et al. Aripiprazole monotherapy for maintenance therapy in bipolar I disorder: a 100-week, double-blind study versus placebo. *J Clin Psychiatry*. 2007;68:1480-1491.

121 Vieta E, Parramon G, Padrell E, et al. Quetiapine in the treatment of rapid cycling bipolar disorder. *Bipolar Disord*. 2002;4:335-340.

122 Vieta E. Mood stabilization in the treatment of bipolar disorder: focus on quetiapine. *Hum Psychopharmacol*. 2005;20:225-236.

123 Vieta E, Suppes T, Eggens I, et al. Efficacy and safety of quetiapine in combination with lithium or divalproex for maintenance of patients with bipolar I disorder (International trial 126). *J Affect Disord*. 2008;109:251-263.

124 Suppes T, Vieta E, Liu S, et al; Trial 127 Investigators. Maintenance treatment for patients with bipolar I disorder: results from a North American study of quetiapine in combination with lithium or divalproex (Trial 127). *Am J Psychiatry*. 2009;166:476-488.

125 Weisler RH, Nolen WA, Neijber A, et al; Trial 144 Study Investigators. Continuation of quetiapine versus switching to placebo or lithium for maintenance treatment of bipolar I disorder (Trial 144: a randomized controlled study). *J Clin Psychiatry* 2011; 72:1452-1464.

126 Macfadden W, Alphs L, Haskins JT, et al. A randomized, double-blind, placebo-controlled study of maintenance treatment with adjunctive risperidone long-acting therapy in patients with bipolar I disorder who relapse frequently. *Bipolar Disord*. 2009;11:827-839.

127 Vieta E, Nieto E, Autet A, et al. A long-term prospective study on the outcome of bipolar patients treated with long-acting injectable risperidone. *World J Biol Psychiatry.* 2008;23:1-6.

128 Vieta E, Goikolea JM. Atypical antipsychotics: newer options for mania and maintenance therapy. *Bipolar Disord.* 2005; 7(suppl 4):21-33.

129 Popovic D, Reinares M, Goikoles JM, et al. Polarity index of pharmacological agents used for maintenance treatment of bipolar disorder. *Eur Neuropsychopharmacol.* 2012;22:339-346.

Chapter 9

Treatment-resistant bipolar disorder

Refractory mania

There are a number of options available for patients with acute mania who have failed to respond to adequate trials of established first- and second-line therapies. Add-on or experimental therapies that are reported to have antimanic activity include phenytoin, levetiracetam, mexiletine, omega-3 fatty acids, oxcarbazepine, rapid tryptophan depletion, allopurinol, amisulphide, and calcitonin [1]. There are also a few studies with standard antimanic agents in the treatment-resistant population.

Electroconvulsive treatment (ECT) may be considered in patients with severe or treatment-resistant mania. A literature review concluded that ECT was effective, particularly in patients who responded poorly to pharmacotherapy, and brought about remission or marked clinical improvement in up to 80% of patients [2]. However, the authors were unable to draw conclusions with respect to relapse, the effect on cognition, and the comparative merits of unilateral versus bilateral ECT. In a separate review of therapeutic trials, the best responses occurred in patients who received a series of nine ECT treatments followed by lithium maintenance [3].

Other emerging non-pharmacological options include transcranial magnetic stimulation (TMS) and vagal nerve stimulation. One controlled trial of repetitive TMS in mania demonstrated that stimulation of the right prefrontal cortex produced a greater improvement in mania than left hemisphere stimulation [4]. This study was, however, methodologically

E. Vieta, *Managing Bipolar Disorder in Clinical Practice*,
DOI: 10.1007/978-1-908517-94-4_9, © Springer Healthcare 2013

weakened by the absence of a sham-treated control group. There are also reports of TMS-induced hypomania [5].

Tamoxifen has been reported to be extremely effective in mania [6,7], but its characteristics make it unsuitable for regular manic episodes. It should be regarded, however, as a potential option for treatment-resistant episodes.

Mixed states

Mixed states are, by definition, difficult to treat. Dysphoric mania may respond to valproate, olanzapine, ziprasidone, or aripiprazole, and to several combinations [8], but much less evidence is available with regard to mixed depressions. Electroconvulsive treatment may be particularly useful in patients with treatment-resistant mixed episodes [9], in whom the risk of switching into depression can be extremely high [10].

Chronic depression

The management of bipolar disorder patients in whom the predominant feature is recurrent depressive episodes has been described as 'extraordinarily understudied' [11]. The treatment of acute, treatment-refractory bipolar depression is complex, with few evidence-based trials [12,13]. In 2009, Pacchiarotti et al proposed new operational criteria for resistance in bipolar depression. They suggest separate criteria for bipolar I and bipolar II resistance [12]:

- Bipolar I: depressive episode that fails to reach remission with adequately dosed lithium (0.8 mEq/L in the plasma) or to other adequate ongoing mood-stabilizing treatment, plus lamotrigine 50–200 mg/day or greater than 600 mg/day of quetiapine as monotherapy.
- Bipolar II: depressive episode that fails to reach remission with adequately dosed lithium (0.8 mEq/L in the plasma) or to other adequate ongoing mood-stabilizing treatment, plus lamotrigine 50–200 mg/day or 300–600 mg/day of quetiapine as monotherapy.

When first and second options fail, the most effective alternative is again ECT [11]. A trial designed to assess the efficacy and safety of ECT for treatment-resistant depression compared with pharmacological therapies is currently ongoing. Patients will be initially randomized to ECT or drug treatment for 6 weeks and then will be given maintenance therapy of the investigator's choice for an additional 20 weeks [14]. The study is expected to be completed in 2013.

Potential options for the pharmacological treatment of refractory depressive episodes include combinations of agents such as quetiapine, lamotrigine, olanzapine, lithium, and valproate with antidepressants, and also agents such as pramipexole or modafinil [15–17]. Since glutathione depletion is a feature of depression and bipolar disorder, add-on treatment with N-acetyl cysteine, its acetylated derivative, may be helpful in reducing depressive symptoms [18].

Vagal nerve stimulation may be effective in bipolar patients with long-lasting, chronic, treatment-resistant depressive episodes, although the evidence base is very limited [19].

Rapid cycling

Patients who have experienced four or more episodes of depression, mania, mixed state, or hypomania in the preceding 12 months are classified as showing rapid cycling. The lifetime risk of rapid cycling in bipolar disorder is around 13–20% [20]; it tends to develop late in the course of the disorder, and is commonly associated with the female gender and bipolar II disorder [21].

Secondary causes of rapid cycling include subclinical hypothyroidism (sometimes lithium induced), substance misuse, and medical comorbidities (eg, sleep apnea, multiple sclerosis, head injury) [20].

Rapid cycling obviously implies temporal severity and can be difficult to treat. It is generally accepted that rapid cycling predicts a poor response to lithium, but this may be the case for all sorts of therapy. In 30–40% of cases, rapid cycling is preceded by exposure to antidepressants, and exacerbated by antidepressant therapy, although there is no proof of causal relationship [21].

The management of rapid cycling involves, in the first instance, careful evaluation of the patient for possible substance abuse and comorbid medical conditions. Where relevant, antidepressant drugs should be gradually tapered and discontinued. Treatment should then be directed at establishing a mood-stabilizing regimen that eliminates cycle-promoting agents, and adds or optimizes treatments with mood-stabilizing properties.

There are few controlled treatment trials in patients with rapid cycling. However, the limited available evidence supports to some extent the use of valproate [22], olanzapine [23,24], lamotrigine [25,26], quetiapine [27,28], risperidone [29], aripiprazole [30], ziprasidone [31], oxcarbazepine in combination with lithium [32], or adjunctive gabapentin [33]. The calcium antagonist nimodipine has also been found to be effective in previously refractory bipolar I disorder, rapid cycling patients [34]. Other experimental therapies are chromium and retigabine [35,36].

Specific, randomized, double-blind trials focused on rapid cyclers are rare. One such trial compared valproate with lithium monotherapy [37] and contrary to what was expected, there were no differences between valproate and lithium with regard to efficacy. Remarkably, only a minority of patients achieved remission during the open-label phase and were able to be randomized for maintenance treatment. Lamotrgine was also specifically studied in rapid cycling with some positive outcome in secondary analysis in bipolar II disorder patients [25].

Additionally, the combination of lithium and carbamazepine, valproate, or lamotrigine for maintenance has some support from controlled studies, as does the adjunctive use of olanzapine [38,39]. Maintenance ECT may also be considered in selected cases [20].

The treatment of rapid cycling requires, for most cases, combinations of several drugs. However, the potential efficacy enhancement has to be balanced with the risk of interactions and increased side effects, particularly the cognitive ones [40].

References

1   Yatham LN, Kennedy SH, Schaffer A, et al. Canadian Network for Mood and Anxiety Treatments (CANMAT) and International Society for Bipolar Disorders (ISBD) collaborative update of CANMAT guidelines for the management of patients with bipolar disorder: update 2009. *Bipolar Disord.* 2009;11:225-255.

2   Mukherjee S, Sackeim HA, Schnurr DB. Electroconvulsive therapy of acute manic episodes: a review of 50 years' experience. *Am J Psychiatry.* 1994;151:169-176.

3   Small JG, Klapper MH, Milstein V, et al. Comparison of therapeutic modalities for mania. *Psychopharmacol Bull.* 1996; 32:623-627.

4   Grisaru N, Chudakov B, Yaroslavsky Y, et al. Transcranial magnetic stimulation in mania: a controlled study. *Am J Psychiatry*. 1998;155:1608-1610.

5   Garcia-Toro M. Acute manic symptomatology during repetitive transcranial magnetic stimulation in a patient with bipolar depression. *Br J Psychiatry*. 1999;175:491.

6   Zarate CA Jr, Singh JB, Carlson PJ, et al. Efficacy of a protein kinase C inhibitor (tamoxifen) in the treatment of acute mania: a pilot study. *Bipolar Disord*. 2007;9:561-70.

7   Yildiz A, Guleryuz S, Ankerst DP, et al. Protein kinase C inhibition in the treatment of mania: a double-blind, placebo-controlled trial of tamoxifen. *Arch Gen Psychiatry*. 2008;65:255-263.

8   Vieta E. Bipolar mixed states and their treatment. *Expert Rev Neurother*. 2005;5:63-68.

9   Valentí M, Benabarre A, García-Amador M, et al. Electroconvulsive therapy in the treatment of mixed states in bipolar disorder. *Eur Psychiatry*. 2008;23:53-56.

10   Vieta E. The treatment of mixed states and the risk of switching to depression. *Eur Psychiatry*. 2005;20:96-100.

11   Valentí M, Benabarre A, Bernardo M, et al. Electroconvulsive therapy in the treatment of bipolar depression. *Actas Esp Psiquiatr*. 2007;35:199-207.

12   Pacchiarotti I, Mazzarini L, Colom F, et al. Treatment-resistant bipolar depression: towards a new definition. *Acta Psychiatr Scand*. 2009;120:429-440.

13   Vieta E, Colom F. Therapeutic options in treatment-resistant depression. *Ann Med*. 2011;43:512-530.

14   Kessler U, Vaaler AE, Schøyen H, et al. The study protocol of the Norwegian randomized controlled trial of electroconvulsive therapy in treatment resistant depression in bipolar disorder. *BMC Psychiatry*. 2010;10:16.

15   Vieta E, Rosa AR. Evolving trends in the long-term treatment of bipolar disorder. *World J Biol Psychiatry*. 2007;8:4-11.

16   Goldberg JF, Burdick KE, Endick CJ. Preliminary randomized, double-blind, placebo-controlled trial of pramipexole added to mood stabilizers for treatment-resistant bipolar depression. *Am J Psychiatry*. 2004;161:564-566.

17   Frye MA, Grunze H, Suppes T, et al. A placebo-controlled evaluation of adjunctive modafinil in the treatment of bipolar depression. *Am J Psychiatry*. 2007;164:1242-1249.

18   Berk M, Copolov DL, Dean O, et al. N-acetyl cysteine for depressive symptoms in bipolar disorder-a double-blind randomized placebo-controlled trial. *Biol Psychiatry*. 2008;64:468-475.

19   Daban C, Martinez-Aran A, Cruz N, et al. Safety and efficacy of Vagus Nerve Stimulation in treatment-resistant depression. A systematic review. *J Affect Disord*. 2008;110:1-15.

20   Vieta E. *Managing the Rapid-Cycling Patient*. London, UK: Nowpharma; 2007.

21   Calabrese JR, Shelton MD, Rapport DJ, et al. Current research on rapid cycling bipolar disorder and its treatment. *J Affect Disord*. 2001;67:241-255.

22   Calabrese JR, Rapport DJ, Kimmel SE, et al. Rapid cycling bipolar disorder and its treatment with valproate. *Can J Psychiatry*. 1993;38(suppl 2):S57-S61.

23   Sanger TM, Tohen M, Vieta E, et al. Olanzapine in the acute treatment of bipolar I disorder with a history of rapid cycling. *J Affect Disord*. 2003;73:155-161.

24   Vieta E, Calabrese JR, Hennen J, et al. Comparison of rapid-cycling and non-rapid-cycling bipolar I manic patients during treatment with olanzapine: analysis of pooled data. *J Clin Psychiatry*. 2004;65:1420-1428.

25   Calabrese J, Suppes T, Bowden C et al. A double-blind, placebo-controlled, prophylaxis study of lamotrigine in rapid-cycling bipolar disorder. Lamictal 614 Study Group. *J Clin Psychiatry*. 2000;61:841-850.

26   Frye M, Ketter T, Kimbrell T, et al. A placebo-controlled study of lamotrigine and gabapentin monotherapy in refractory mood disorders. *J Clin Psychopharmacol*. 2000;20:607-614.

27   Vieta E, Parramon G, Padrell E, et al. Quetiapine in the treatment of rapid cycling bipolar disorder. *Bipolar Disord*. 2002;4:335-340.

28 Vieta E, Calabrese JR, Goikolea JM, et al. Quetiapine monotherapy in the treatment of patients with bipolar I or II depression and a rapid-cycling disease course: a randomized, double-blind, placebo-controlled study. *Bipolar Disord*. 2007;9:413-425.

29 Vieta E, Gasto C, Colom F, et al; BOLDER Study Group. Treatment of refractory rapid cycling bipolar disorder with risperidone. *J Clin Psychopharmacol*. 1998;18:172-174.

30 Muzina DJ, Momah C, Eudicone JM, et al. Aripiprazole monotherapy in patients with rapid-cycling bipolar I disorder: an analysis from a long-term, double-blind, placebo-controlled study. *Int J Clin Pract*. 2008;62:679-687.

31 Fountoulakis KN, Vieta E, Siamouli M, et al. Treatment of bipolar disorder: a complex treatment for a multi-faceted disorder. *Ann Gen Psychiatry*. 2007;6:27.

32 Vieta E, Cruz N, García-Campayo J, et al. A double-blind, randomized, placebo-controlled prophylaxis trial of oxcarbazepine as adjunctive treatment to lithium in the long-term treatment of bipolar I and II disorder. *Int J Neuropsychopharmacol*. 2008;11:445-452.

33 Vieta E, Manuel GJ, Martinez-Aran A, et al. A double-blind, randomized, placebo-controlled, prophylaxis study of adjunctive gabapentin for bipolar disorder. *J Clin Psychiatry*. 2006;67:473-477.

34 Pazzaglia PJ, Post RM, Ketter TA, et al. Nimodipine monotherapy and carbamazepine augmentation in patients with refractory recurrent affective illness. *J Clin Psychopharmacol*. 1998;18:404-413.

35 Amann BL, Mergl R, Vieta E, et al. A 2-year, open-label pilot study of adjunctive chromium in patients with treatment-resistant rapid-cycling bipolar disorder. *J Clin Psychopharmacol*. 2007;27:104-106.

36 Amann B, Sterr A, Vieta E, et al. An exploratory open trial on safety and efficacy of the anticonvulsant retigabine in acute manic patients. *J Clin Psychopharmacol*. 2006;26:534-536.

37 Calabrese JR, Shelton MD, Rapport DJ, et al. A 20-month, double-blind, maintenance trial of lithium versus divalproex in rapid-cycling bipolar disorder. *Am J Psychiatry*. 2005;162:2152-2161.

38 Coryell W. Rapid cycling bipolar disorder: clinical characteristics and treatment options. *CNS Drugs*. 2005;19:557-569.

39 Cruz N, Vieta E, Comes M, et al; the EMBLEM Advisory Board. Rapid-cycling bipolar I disorder: Course and treatment outcome of a large sample across Europe. *J Psychiatr Res*. 2008;42:1068-1075.

40 Martinez-Aran A, Vieta E, Colom F, et al. Do cognitive complaints in euthymic bipolar patients reflect objective cognitive impairment? *Psychother Psychosom*. 2005;74:295-302.

Chapter 10

Psychosocial interventions

Although pharmacotherapy is the mainstay of treatment for bipolar disorder, it is now widely recognized that specific psychosocial interventions (beyond regular monitoring and supportive care) offer additional benefits for the patient, family, and caregivers.

Several methodologically sound trials have demonstrated that adjunctive psychosocial approaches improve the overall effectiveness of treatment, mainly through further protection against relapse or recurrence, and this findings were backed up by a meta-analysis of 19 trials [1–3]. Other targets of psychosocial intervention include social functioning, subsyndromal symptoms, treatment adherence, hospitalization, need for medications, psychiatric comorbidity, biological rhythms, and prodrome recognition.

Reflecting this growing body of evidence, most treatment guidelines now endorse psychosocial treatments as sensible add-on choices [4,5], especially in the maintenance phase of treatment of bipolar spectrum illnesses, and four such approaches are described below. Table 10.1 lists the potential mediators that could explain the positive effects of psychosocial treatments on outcomes in bipolar disorder [3].

Cognitive–behavioral therapy

Cognitive–behavioral therapy (CBT) focuses on the interaction of disordered thinking, mood, and behavior. Patients are taught to monitor and change automatic, dysfunctional thinking and behaviors that arise

E. Vieta, *Managing Bipolar Disorder in Clinical Practice*,
DOI: 10.1007/978-1-908517-94-4_10, © Springer Healthcare 2013

Potential mediators of the effects of adjunctive psychotherapy on illness outcomes in bipolar disorder

- Acquiring emotional self-regulation skills
- Acquiring balanced and less pessimistic attitudes toward the self in relation to the illness
- Improving family relationships and communication
- Improving social skills
- Decreasing self-stigmatization and increasing acceptance of the disorder
- Increasing external social and treatment supports
- Enhancing medication adherence
- Stabilizing sleep/wake cycles and other daily routines
- Improving ability to identify and intervene early with relapses

Table 10.1 Potential mediators of the effects of adjunctive psychotherapy on illness outcomes in bipolar disorder. Reproduced with permission from Miklowitz et al [3].

from their mood states, thereby improving coping mechanisms and social functioning.

CBT has been evaluated in several well-designed studies. A preliminary, small, randomized controlled pilot study showed that patients who received 6 months of CBT had more improvement in depressive symptomatology and functioning than controls [6]. Subsequently, a few further studies have assessed CBT in bipolar depression and in maintenance [7–10]. One of the largest studies could not prove any advantage of CBT over treatment as usual on relapse rates [8]. CBT was even harmful in patients who had experienced 12 or more episodes in their lifetime [8]. A possible explanation is that the patients who are more euthymic are more likely to benefit from the educational component of the intervention [11].

Another randomized controlled trial found that patients who received 12 months of group CBT in conjunction with their regular medications had significantly fewer depressive and manic episodes, days experiencing an episode, and number of hospital admissions compared with patients who received medication only [9]. The CBT group also had significantly higher social functioning and better adherence to medication.

However, continued observation of this cohort suggested that the benefits of CBT decreased over time [10]. After 30 months of follow-up, the CBT group had significantly better outcomes in terms of time to relapse, but the benefit mainly occurred in the first year. The authors suggest that, as therapy became more distant, the benefits became weaker, suggesting a need to explore the use of booster sessions or maintenance psychotherapy. The weakening of the positive benefits may offset the cost advantages of using CBT over the long term [12]. In summary, there is conflicting evidence supporting the use of CBT in bipolar disorder. A possible explanation is that only the behavioral and educational components of the CBT packages in the mentioned studies were actually active, and perhaps the cognitive component may be less relevant as emotions may preclude cognition in bipolar illness [11,13].

Psychoeducation

Psychoeducation aims to provide patients with a theoretical and practical approach to understanding and coping with the consequences of their illness. Psychoeducation is founded on a medical model. The primary goals of psychoeducation are to reduce rates of relapse and hospitalization, and improve functional outcomes by enhancing illness awareness, promoting early detection of prodromal symptoms, increasing medication adherence, and preventing suicidal behavior. Other aspects of psychoeducation include promoting healthy sleeping habits as a tool to prevent relapse, and improving patients' overall quality of life by reducing stigma and guilt, increasing self-esteem and well-being, reducing comorbidities, and avoiding a stress-inducing lifestyle [14]. Psychoeducation is best implemented when the patient is euthymic and less likely to have dysfunctional symptoms [12].

Various psychoeducational approaches have proved effective in clinical studies. In a single-blind controlled study, 69 patients with a relapse in the previous 12 months were randomized to routine care alone or with 7–12 individual sessions with a psychologist [15]. Patients were taught to recognize their own prodromal symptoms and to seek prompt medical attention when they occurred. Compared with routine care, patients who also received psychoeducation had a significantly longer time to manic episodes, fewer manic episodes, and overall improvements in social functioning and employment. The intervention had no effect on depressive episodes.

Group psychoeducation has also been found to be effective in preventing recurrences. The treatment protocol developed by the Barcelona Bipolar Disorders Program involves groups of 8–12 euthymic patients directed by two trained psychologists, in 21 weekly 90-minute sessions. The contents of the program are shown in Table 10.2 [16]. A randomized controlled study of this approach found that it significantly reduced the time to recurrence of both manic and depressive episodes, as well as the number of recurrences per patient, compared with the control group [16].

There were an additional three years of follow-up to the original 2-year study period; survival curves of time to recurrence over the entire 5 years are shown in Figure 10.1. Thirty percent of patients in the treatment group required hospitalization compared with 40% of the control group [17]. Patients in the treatment group had significantly better social and occupational functioning after 5 years (*P*<0.006) [18].

The efficacy of psychoeducation is not solely related to improvement of compliance [19]. In a subsequent study, highly adherent patients also showed benefit from psychoeducation in prevention of further recurrences of illness [20]. As noted above, psychoeducation proved useful to prevent manic, hypomanic, mixed, and depressive recurrences during

Contents of the psychoeducative program (Barcelona Bipolar Disorders Program)

1. Introduction
2. What is bipolar illness?
3. Causal and triggering factors
4. Symptoms (I): mania and hypomania
5. Symptoms (II): depression and mixed episodes
6. Course and outcome
7. Treatment (I): mood stabilisers
8. Treatment (II): antimanic agents
9. Treatment (III): antidepressants
10. Serum levels: lithium, carbamazepine, and valproate
11. Pregnancy and genetic counselling
12. Psychopharmacology vs alternative therapies
13. Risks associated with treatment withdrawal
14. Alcohol and street drugs: risks in bipolar illness
15. Early detection of manic and hypomanic episodes
16. Early detection of depressive and mixed episodes
17. What to do when a new phase is detected
18. Lifestyle regularity
19. Stress management techniques
20. Problem-solving techniques
21. Final session

Table 10.2 Contents of the psychoeducative program (Barcelona Bipolar Disorders Program). Reproduced from Colom et al [16].

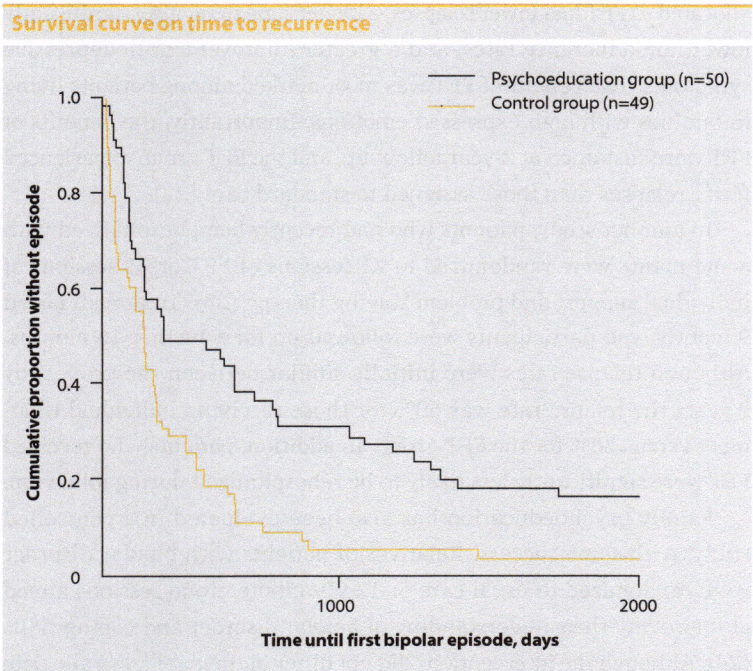

Figure 10.1 Survival curve on time to recurrence. Reproduced with permission from Colom et al [17].

a 5-year follow-up after a 6-month group intervention [17]. The results were also positive when the bipolar II disorder subgroup was analyzed separately [18].

Family-focused therapy

Family-focused therapy (FFT) is similar to psychoeducation, but places greater emphasis on achieving the support and cooperation of family and caregivers as integral components of successful treatment. The goal of FFT is to improve family functioning through training in communication, problem-solving and coping strategies, psychoeducation, and relapse prevention techniques.

A total of 21 sessions of adjunctive FFT was compared with the usual care plus a brief, two-session family intervention in a randomized controlled study [21]. Compared with the brief intervention, patients allocated to FFT had fewer relapses, a longer time to relapse, significantly lower non-adherence rates, and a greater improvement in depressive symptoms. The benefit of FFT was most marked among patients living in families with high expressed emotions. Importantly, the benefits of FFT were sustained at 2-year follow-up, and the FFT group experienced fewer relapses than those assigned to standard care [22].

In another study, patients who had recently been hospitalized with acute mania were randomized to 21 sessions of FFT or 21 sessions of individual support and problem-solving therapy [23]. Treatment lasted 9 months and participants were followed up for a further 15 months. Although relapse rates were initially similar between the groups, by 2 years the relapse rate was 60% for those receiving individual treatment versus 28% for the FFT group. In addition, patients who received FFT were significantly less likely to be rehospitalized during follow-up.

Family psychoeducation has also been evaluated in a controlled study, with some success. Relatives of patients with bipolar disorder were randomized to usual care or 12 90-minute group sessions aimed at improving their understanding of bipolar disorder and coping skills [24]. Although the interventions did not differ in their ability to alleviate the objective burden, psychoeducated caregivers showed a significant improvement in their knowledge of bipolar disorder and a reduction in the subjective burden. During the course of the sessions, blame on the patient increased in the control group but fell in the psychoeducation group (Figure 10.2) [24].

The efficacy of family psychoeducation has been further supported by other recent studies [7,24,25]. The only trial that looked at the outcome of bipolar disorder patients whose caregivers had received family psychoeducation showed a significant impact on the prevention of mania but not depression [26], suggesting that relatives and partners may be better at detecting early signs of mania than depression.

A staging model may be helpful in improving outcomes with FFT and assisting with treatment prognosis [27]. In a recent study, 113 patients with bipolar disorders were divided into Stage I (no impairment and well-established euthymia) and Stages II-IV, or 'advanced stages' (increasing levels of cognitive and functional impairment), and were further defined

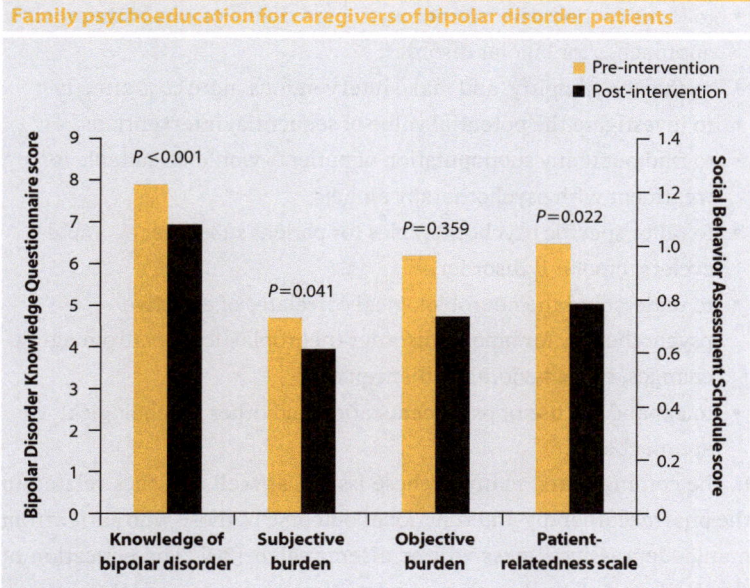

Figure 10.2 Family psychoeducation for caregivers of bipolar disorder patients. Reproduced with permission from Reinares et al [24].

by treatment and control. Patients in Stage I whose caregivers have had psychoeducation had the fewest rates of recurrence [28].

Interpersonal and social rhythm therapy

There is some evidence that this type of therapy may be helpful for bipolar disorder patients, particularly for those with medical comorbidities [7,29]. Sleep and social activity are important targets of this sort of intervention and the potential mechanism of action may well be basically behavioral.

The challenges for the future in the area of bipolar disorder psycho-therapy are:

- to develop effective psychotherapies for hypomanic and mixed episodes;
- to integrate the prevention of physical comorbidities and mortality into the therapy by promoting healthy habits during psychoeducative interventions;
- to integrate cognitive remediation into psychotherapy programs;

- to identify the active and common ingredients of psychotherapeutic approaches for bipolar disorder;
- to shorten, simplify, and make interventions more cost-effective;
- to investigate the potential value of sequential interventions;
- to find out if any subpopulation of patients would be suitable for treatment with psychotherapy alone;
- to tailor specific psychotherapies for patient subtypes (eg, rapid cyclers, bipolar II disorder);
- to understand the neurobiological correlates of effective psychotherapy for bipolar disorder (neuroplasticity, neuroimaging changes, biobehavioral resilience); and
- to expand the use of psychoeducation and other psychological approaches.

In the coming years, many of these issues, as well as issues related to the pharmacotherapy and functional outcome of those who suffer from manic–depressive illness will be disentangled [30]. The education of clinicians and all the key players in health care may be crucial to achieve a good outcome.

References

1   Vieta E, Pacchiarotti I, Scott J, et al. Evidence-based research on the efficacy of psychologic interventions in bipolar disorders: a critical review. *Curr Psychiatry Rep*. 2005;7:449-455.
2   Vieta E, Colom F. Psychological interventions in bipolar disorder: From wishful thinking to an evidence-based approach. *Acta Psychiatr Scand Suppl*. 2004;34-38.
3   Miklowitz DJ, Scott J. Psychosocial treatments for bipolar disorder: cost-effectiveness, mediating mechanisms, and future directions. *Bipolar Disord*. 2009;11(suppl 2):110-122.
4   Fountoulakis KN, Vieta E, Sanchez-Moreno J, et al. Treatment guidelines for bipolar disorder: a critical review. *J Affect Disord*. 2005;86:1-10.
5   Yatham LN, Kennedy SH, Schaffer A, et al. Canadian Network for Mood and Anxiety Treatments (CANMAT) and International Society for Bipolar Disorders (ISBD) collaborative update of CANMAT guidelines for the management of patients with bipolar disorder: update 2009. *Bipolar Disord*. 2009;11:225-255.
6   Scott J, Garland A, Moorhead S. A pilot study of cognitive therapy in bipolar disorders. *Psychol Med*. 2001;31:459-467.
7   Miklowitz DJ, Otto MW, Frank E, et al. Psychosocial treatments for bipolar depression: a 1-year randomized trial from the Systematic Treatment Enhancement Program. *Arch Gen Psychiatry*. 2007;64:419-426.
8   Scott J, Paykel E, Morriss R, et al. Cognitive-behavioural therapy for severe and recurrent bipolar disorders: randomised controlled trial. *Br J Psychiatry*. 2006;188:313-320.
9   Lam DH, Watkins ER, Hayward P, et al. A randomized controlled study of cognitive therapy for relapse prevention for bipolar affective disorder: outcome of the first year. *Arch Gen Psychiatry*. 2003;60:145-152.

10 Lam DH, Hayward P, Watkins ER, et al. Relapse prevention in patients with bipolar disorder: cognitive therapy outcome after 2 years. *Am J Psychiatry*. 2005;162:324-329.

11 Scott J, Colom F, Vieta E. A meta-analysis of relapse rates with adjunctive psychological therapies compared to usual psychiatric treatment for bipolar disorders. *Int J Neuropsychopharmacol*. 2007;10:123-129.

12 Vieta E, Pacchiarotti I, Valentí M, et al. A critical update on psychological interventions for bipolar disorder. *Curr Psychiatry Rep*. 2009;11:494-502.

13 Colom F, Vieta E. Sudden glory revisited: cognitive contents of hypomania. *Psychother Psychosom*. 2007; 76:278-288.

14 Colom F, Vieta E. *Psychoeducation Manual for Bipolar Disorder*. Cambridge, UK: Cambridge University Press; 2006.

15 Perry A, Tarrier N, Morriss R, et al. Randomised controlled trial of efficacy of teaching patients with bipolar disorder to identify early symptoms of relapse and obtain treatment. *BMJ*. 1999;318:149-153.

16 Colom F, Vieta E, Martinez-Aran A, et al. A randomized trial on the efficacy of group psychoeducation in the prophylaxis of recurrences in bipolar patients whose disease is in remission. *Arch Gen Psychiatry*. 2003;60:402-407.

17 Colom F, Vieta E, Sánchez-Moreno J, et al. Group psychoeducation for stabilised bipolar disorders: 5-year outcome of a randomised clinical trial. *Br J Psychiatry*. 2009;194:260-265.

18 Colom F, Vieta E, Sánchez-Moreno J, et al. Psychoeducation for bipolar II disorder: an exploratory, 5-year outcome subanalysis. *J Affect Disord*. 2009;112:30-35.

19 Vieta E. Improving treatment adherence in bipolar disorder through psychoeducation. *J Clin Psychiatry*. 2005;66(suppl 1):24-29.

20 Colom F, Vieta E, Reinares M et al. Psychoeducation efficacy in bipolar disorders: beyond compliance enhancement. J Clin Psychiatry. 2003; 64:1101-1105.

21 Miklowitz DJ, Simoneau TL, George EL, et al. Family-focused treatment of bipolar disorder: 1-year effects of a psychoeducational program in conjunction with pharmacotherapy. *Biol Psychiatry*. 2000;48:582-592.

22 Miklowitz DJ, George EL, Richards JA, et al. A randomized study of family-focused psychoeducation and pharmacotherapy in the outpatient management of bipolar disorder. *Arch Gen Psychiatry*. 2003;60:904-912.

23 Rea MM, Tompson MC, Miklowitz DJ, et al. Family-focused treatment versus individual treatment for bipolar disorder: results of a randomized clinical trial. *J Consult Clin Psychol*. 2003;71:482-492.

24 Reinares M, Vieta E, Colom F, et al. Impact of a psychoeducational family intervention on caregivers of stabilized bipolar patients. *Psychother Psychosom*. 2004;73:312-319.

25 Miklowitz DJ, Otto MW, Frank E, et al. Intensive psychosocial intervention enhances functioning in patients with bipolar depression: results from a 9-month randomized controlled trial. *Am J Psychiatry*. 2007;164:1340-1347.

26 Reinares M, Colom F, Sánchez-Moreno J, et al. Impact of caregiver group psychoeducation on the course and outcome of bipolar patients in remission: a randomized controlled trial. *Bipolar Disord*. 2008;10:511-519.

27 Vieta E, Reinares M, Rosa AR. Staging bipolar disorder. *Neurotox Res*. 2011;19:279-285.

28 Reinares M, Colom F, Rosa AR, et al. The impact of staging bipolar disorder on treatment outcome of family psychoeducation. *J Affect Disord*. 2010;123:81-86.

29 Frank E, Kupfer DJ, Thase ME, et al. Two-year outcomes for interpersonal and social rhythm therapy in individuals with bipolar I disorder. *Arch Gen Psychiatry*. 2005;62:996-1004.

30 Vieta E, Rosa AR. Evolving trends in the long-term treatment of bipolar disorder. *World J Biol Psychiatry*. 2007;8:4-11.